Nisei Cadet Nurse
of
WORLD WAR II

Patriotism in Spite of Prejudice

THELMA M. ROBINSON

Black Swan Mill Press
BOULDER, COLORADO

ISBN: 0-615-13022-4
Library of Congress Control Number: 2005909681

Japanese translations and calligraphy by Takeko Nishida
Book design and typesetting by Troy Scott Parker, Cimarron Design,
   cimarrondesign.com
Printed in the United States of America

Address inquiries to:
   Black Swan Mill Press
   2525 Arapahoe Ave., Suite E4
   PMB 534
   Boulder, CO 80302 USA

For further information:
   www.cadetnurse.com

Cover photo:
   Nisei Cadet Nurses in student uniform, St. Mary's Hospital School of Nursing, Rochester, Minnesota, 1945. Top: Mary (Izumi) Tamura. Middle, left to right: Mary (Sagata) Tamura, Ida (Sakohira) Kawaguchi. Bottom: Sharon (Tanagi) Aburano. Photo courtesy Sharon Aburano and Ida Kawaguchi.

Back cover photos:
   [Top] Heart Mountain Relocation Camp. Photo courtesy of American Heritage Center, University of Wyoming.
   [Left center] Grace Obata Amemiya, one of the first two Nisei women ever accepted for affiliation as a senior cadet in the Army Nurse Corps, 1945. Photo courtesy Grace Amemiya.
   [Right center] Cadet Nurse uniform shoulder badge.

From 1943 to 1948, the U.S. Cadet Nurse Corps
was the largest and youngest group of uniformed women
to serve in World War II

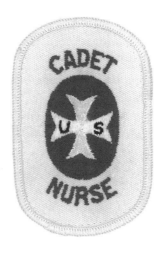

The Maltese cross, once worn by the Knights of St. John, survived the crusades and became the insignia of many groups caring for the sick. It was on the banner of the U.S. Cadet Nurse Corps and was worn on the shoulders of the nurse's uniform. The eight points of the cross signify the beatitudes:

Spiritual joy
To live without malice
To weep over thy sins
To humble thyself
To love justice
To be merciful
To be sincere and pure of heart
To suffer persecution

Source:
M. Patricia Donahue, *Nursing The Finest Art: An Illustrated History (second edition)*, (St. Louis, Missouri: Mosby, 1996), 126.

Contents

Acknowledgments

In January of 1999 my sister, Paulie Perry and I, along with former cadet nurses in the San Francisco area, celebrated Lucile Petry Leone's ninety-seventh birthday. (Mrs. Leone died November 25, 1999.) For five years, we cadets of World War II had come together to honor and share memories with Mrs. Leone, Emeritus Director of the U.S. Cadet Nurse Corps. Mrs. Leone had applauded our efforts in documenting cadet nurse stories. The first cadet nurse project was coming to fruition. My concern was that the Japanese American cadet legacy needed to be told in more depth.

I asked Ida Kawaguchi and her husband Masaru, Stella Kato and her husband Yo, and Alice Kanagaki to join me for lunch to discuss the possibility of a future project to tell the story of the Nisei nurse of World War II. This was the beginning; without their enthusiasm, encouragement, and support, this book would never have been written.

Many individuals contributed to the fulfillment of the Nisei Cadet Nurse Project now in book form. First and foremost, I wish to thank the Japanese American women and their families who made major contributions in writing their stories, participating in interviews, and sharing their photographs and other memorabilia. Not only did they offer heartfelt insights regarding their experiences, but they also set about recruiting their peers. This book is dedicated to these women who shared their stories.

The American Association of the History of Nursing (AAHN) has been my foremost inspiration. After more than 40 years of hands-on nursing, my career took another turn—that of becoming a nurse historian. AAHN workshops, presentations, the meeting of enthusiastic

well-known nurse historians, and the opportunity to present my
project for critique were immeasurably helpful. Through AAHN, I met
Marcia L. Dale, Dean of the University of Wyoming School of Nursing,
and she encouraged me to enroll with an enrichment student status at
their university. Dr. Susan McKay's own research was in the same area
and she became my mentor guiding me through the development of the
manuscript. In 2002 I received the AAHN Cadet Nurse Corps Award
for the Nisei Nurse of World War II (at that time a work in progress).
I was encouraged to pursue publication to enable a broader section to
learn about this event in nursing history.

I am indebted to the following archives, museums, and reference col-
lections for their assistance in accessing oral history materials and
documents.: University of Washington Libraries, Seattle, Washington;
Hoover Institution Archives (Margaret Kimball), Stanford University,
Palo Alto, California; American Friends Service Committee Archives
(Jack Sutton), Philadelphia, Pennsylvania; Archives at University of
Colorado Boulder Libraries (David Hays); American Heritage Center,
University of Wyoming, Laramie, Wyoming (Leslie Shores); Utah
State Historical Society, Salt Lake City, Utah; State Historical Society
of Colorado, Denver, Colorado; National Japanese American Historical
Society, San Francisco, California (Judy Hamaguchi); and Japanese
American National Museum, Los Angeles, California.
    The University of Colorado School of Nursing, my alma mater,
sponsored my lecture, "*Justice denied—and redeemed, The plight
of Japanese American nursing students in World War II*," at the
International Seminar Series (2003). Dean Patricia Moritz and Dr.
Marilyn Kraijeck have supported my nursing history research. Other
publicity regarding my project sparked interest and I thank the following people: Silvia Pettem, Boulder County historian for her article,
Wartime nurse preserves peers' history; and Carey Restino, staff writer
for her article, *Homer women in book about W.W.II nurses*.
    This list would not be complete without the mention of the Women
in Military Service for America Memorial and Director Brigadier

General Wilma L. Vaught (Ret.), who personally encouraged me to collect stories regarding the patriotism of Japanese American cadet nurses during World War II.

In bringing this book toward final completion, I am indebted to the following: Margi Bromberg, Gus Tanaka, MD, and Rob Beebe who read the manuscript and offered suggestions; Marti Anderson, local historian with ongoing suggestions; Clara Thomas, my editor, for her skillful guidance; Troy Scott Parker, compositor with expertise in fitting the pieces together and my wonderful supportive family: my sister, Paulie; my children, Dennis, Mary Louise, Larry, and Bruce and their families; and most of all my husband, Dick, for more reasons than I can tell.

  – Thelma M. Robinson
  October 2005

Introduction

UNITED BY A SPIRIT of caring and commitment, women who were cadet nurses during World War II share a bond of patriotism and dedication. Some of these women, Japanese Americans, overcame the indignities of prejudice by proving their loyalty to their country. For many years, their inspiring life stories have been left untold.

The fiftieth year Commemorative Conference of the United States Cadet Nurse Corps held in Bethesda, Maryland, recognized, and honored women who served as cadet nurses during World War II. The United States Public Health Service (USPHS) administered the Cadet Nurse Corps and sponsored the 1994 jubilee celebration. We cadet nurses had come together to celebrate the Nurse Training Act of 1943, the war measure that alleviated the most critical nurse shortage in the history of our country.

At the 1994 conference, Surgeon General Thomas Parran of the USPHS was remembered when he testified before the House Committee on Military Affairs on February 6, 1945. Dr. Parran reported that the U.S. Cadet Nurse Corps was highly successful in the recruitment effort. The most important and immediate function of the Corps had been the replacement of graduate nurses in civilian hospitals with cadet nurses, making it possible for greater numbers of registered nurses to enter the military.[1] Between the years 1943 and 1948, more than 124,000 cadet nurses graduated from 1,250 schools of nursing, forming the largest and youngest group of uniformed women to serve their country during World War II and early post-war years.[2]

Fifty years later, the story of the U.S. Cadet Nurse Corps had almost been forgotten through the pages of time. My sister Paulie

Perry and I, both cadet nurses, decided to make the Corps legacy better known through a cadet nurse nationwide story telling project. We announced our intent through a poster presentation at the fiftieth year Commemorative Conference of the U.S. Cadet Nurse Corps. The cadet nurses enthusiastically endorsed our project and offered to recruit their classmates.[3] More than 2,000 former cadet nurses were contacted. Three hundred eighty women representing 112 schools of nursing from 33 states responded sharing their stories, photographs, and other memorabilia.

We cadet nurses had grown up in the Great Depression, and many of our families could not afford a college education for us. The Corps gave us the opportunity to gain an education and to serve our country in uniform. This was a way "in" for thousands of young women like myself during World War II. At the commemorative celebration, I learned that for more than 350 Japanese American women, the Corps was a way "out."

Elizabeth Lattell McQuale was a cadet nurse at the Protestant Episcopal Hospital School of Nursing in Philadelphia, Pennsylvania. She told me that her school of nursing was one of the few to accept Japanese American women into her school of nursing, making them eligible for the Cadet Nurse Corps program. "My roommate was an American Japanese and a few years older than I," McQuale said. "Her college was interrupted when she and her family were transported to Arizona to serve in a 'concentration camp.' From some of the tales she told me, it was not pleasant. Sandstorms came up; infirmary facilities were meager; sheets were hung to allow privacy for patients."[4]

Mitsu Hasegawa Nakada, a classmate of McQuale's, lived in Alaska as I did at that time, and she agreed to share her story. I sat spellbound as Mitsu's story unfolded. She had been enrolled in the Los Angeles Hospital School of Nursing when World War II broke out. War hysteria engulfed the Pacific Coast. On February 19, 1942, President Franklin Roosevelt signed Executive Order 9066, the document that paved the way for mass evacuation of those with Japanese ancestry from the Pacific States.[5] Mitsu was one of the 110,000 people uprooted from their homes, jobs and schools. Like 60 percent of the evacuees, Mitsu was an American citizen.

I learned more about the Japanese American cadet nurse story in November 1994, when my sister and I hosted a coffee honoring Lucile Petry (now Leone), director of the Cadet Nurse Corps who was then in her nineties and living in San Francisco, California. The purpose of this occasion was to give the cadet nurses of World War II an opportunity to thank Mrs. Leone for her renowned nursing leadership and to tell her how the Cadet Nurse Corps provided us the promised lifetime education. While sharing their stories, two Japanese American ladies had special words of gratitude. For Stella Horita Kato and Ida Sakohira Kawaguchi, the Corps had not only given them their education but their ticket to freedom. Mrs. Leone learned for the first time how the Corps had provided hundreds of Japanese American young women an opportunity to do something useful for their country and to show that they were loyal American citizens.

For the next five years, cadets came together to help Mrs. Leone celebrate her birthday. As the nationwide storytelling project came to fruition, I realized that the story of the Japanese American cadet nurses was unique and needed to be told with more detail. At Mrs. Leone's 97th birthday celebration, I asked my Japanese American friends if they would be interested in sharing their stories.

These women enthusiastically agreed to participate and began recruiting others. One woman contacted the *Pacific Citizen*, the periodical for the Japanese American Citizens League (JACL). An article appeared in the newspaper describing the project and the number of participants grew to 30. These women not only shared their memories but also sent photos and other memorabilia. For many of the women in this book, their desire to be a nurse began at an early age and heightened during their evacuation experience.

Converted fairgrounds and racetracks became temporary assembly centers for evacuees from the proscribed military zones waiting for permanent relocation. Former student nurses, now evacuees, used their experience to give comfort and advice to mothers of newborn babies and worked in makeshift infirmaries. After several months the evacuees, under military guard, boarded the dilapidated trains headed for the relocation centers. Student nurses spent sleepless nights on evacuation trains caring for the bedridden patients. When they reached the hastily built relocation centers that had all the trappings of prison, they continued to serve in nursing capacities, sometimes beyond their training and with only the minimum of supplies and equipment. They did so in a spirit of caring for others.

Some of the women finished their high school education in the bare barracks and began searching for ways to best serve their country. Many took nurse aide training and worked in hospitals. The Japanese American student nurses who lived beyond the military zones were searched for contraband, knives, guns, radios, and flashlights. Many faced prejudices and tolerated those who called them "Japs."

Finally an opportunity came for these Japanese American women, who were American-born and called "Nisei," to join the U.S. Cadet Nurse Corps. For some this meant leaving their families behind barbed wire and striking out alone in an unknown world. The women pioneered the way for others to leave camp and to follow in their footsteps. The Nisei women entered nursing schools in unfamiliar regions of the country far away from their families, but they were sustained by fortitude, family ties, discipline, and companionship with Caucasian cadet nurses. All of these women demonstrated that there were no barriers in giving their best to their patients regardless of race.

The government evacuated the people with Japanese ancestry from the Pacific Coast on the notion that it would be impossible to distinguish the loyal from the disloyal. Without exception, the women participating in this story say that proving their loyalty to the United States was foremost. They signed their pledge of personal commitment to serve as nurses until World War II was won while their families remained interned in desolate camps.

Nisei Cadet Nurse of World War II is a unique collection of stories woven together with archival and library resources. This book presents the human and personal accounts of Japanese American women in their youth, all citizens by birth, who with their families suffered the indignities of false betrayal. Their spirit of caring and their individual commitment as Japanese American nurses proves their loyalty. They made the most of a difficult situation and taught us a lesson in forgiveness. As one Nisei cadet nurse said, "This is my country, good or bad."

References and Notes

[1] Testimony of Thomas Parran, Surgeon General, U.S. Public Health Service, Before the House Committee on Military Affairs. 1945. *Journal of American Medical Association*, 6 February, 1995.

[2] U.S. Federal Security Agency, Public Health Service. 1950. *The U.S. Cadet Nurse Corps 1943-1948*. (Public Health Service Publication No. 38, p. 97). (Washington, D.C.: Government Printing Office).

[3] Thelma M. Robinson and Paulie M. Perry, *Cadet Nurse Stories: The Call and Response of Women During World War II*, Indianapolis, Indiana: Center Nursing Press: 2001):198.

[4] McQuale, Elizabeth Lattell. 1994. Cadet Nurse story telling Project Participant. Boulder, Colorado.

[5] Maddox, Robert J. 1992. *The United States and World War II*, (Boulder, Colorado: Westview Press, 1992):198.

① Latecomers: The Issei

J APANESE IMMIGRANTS, CALLED ISSEI, began arriving in America in 1890 to better their lives.[1] Unlike immigrants from the British Isles, Germany, and other European countries, these relative latecomers could not become citizens of the United States. The Naturalization Act of 1790 limited citizenship to "alien being a white person," and Asians were considered nonwhite. African Americans were granted citizenship during the post-Civil War era, but not until 1952 did Japanese have that privilege.[2]

In 1886 the emperor of Japan lifted the ban on emigration and encouraged it from the most densely populated areas. At that time Japan was suffering from acute overcrowding. The average laborer's wage was 14¢ a per day, so the promise of $1.50 per day in America was attractive, even though a low wage by American standards. In addition to providing much needed farm labor, the Japanese immigrants worked in mines, on the railroads and in private homes as domestics and gardeners. Some established businesses to cater to their countrymen.[3]

The Japanese had a great knowledge of farming. Japan is made up of 3,000 islands with much mountainous land. The Japanese had learned over centuries how to make what little land they owned to be productive.

Realizing the potential of wasted land in California and Oregon, many Japanese became independent farmers.[4] As Japanese immigrants improved their economic status, California farmers and others became envious. Unions barred Japanese from working in some trades. California school boards discussed segregation, and a few implemented it. Editorials appeared in newspapers about the Japanese "problem," with heated arguments that Japanese were threatening the prosperity of the country.[5]

In 1905 the West's anti-Japanese movement was heard in our nation's capitol. The three major political parties—Republicans, Democrats, and Populists—began calling for an end to all Asian immigration. As Japan was rising to strong military power, President Theodore Roosevelt did not want to offend Japanese leaders by closing the country to Japanese immigrants. Roosevelt took a more subtle approach in settling the problem, negotiating with Japan the "Gentleman's Agreement of 1908." Under these terms the Japanese would stop issuing passports to laborers and limit immigration to the family of those laborers already in America. In return, the United States would stop passing anti-Japanese legislation and would allow limited immigration to continue.[6]

The Gentleman's Agreement increased rather than decreased the number of Japanese coming to the West Coast. Many Japanese immigrants had left wives and families when they came to America. Now many had a legal right to enter the country, and tens of thousands of them did so. Unmarried Japanese men returned to Japan to marry and brought their new wives to the States. But many could not afford the passage back to Japan. Parent-arranged marriages were a common practice in Japan, so women were married by proxy to men they had never seen. A friend of the family would stand in for the groom; then the new bride would set sail for America to join her husband. The majority of the Japanese women, over 33,000 immigrants, entered the United States between 1908 and 1924. Their arrival marked the beginning of Japanese American families.[7]

Author Yoshiko Uchida's mother was a picture bride. She had never met her future husband, but the two had corresponded for more than a year. Both had been students at different times at the Doshisho University in Kyoto, one of Japan's foremost Christian universities. A professor who knew both parties suggested that they write to one another. Uchida reflected:

> I believe those early Issei women must have had tremendous reserves of strength and courage to do what they did, often masked by their quiet and unassertive demeanor. They came to an alien land, created homes for the men, worked beside them in fields, small shops and businesses, and at the same time bore most of the responsibility for raising the

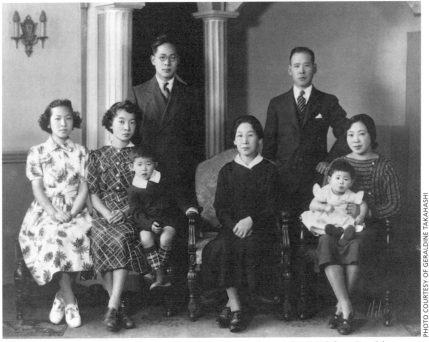

Takahashi family portrait taken in Seattle, 1939. Left to right: Hideko, Geraldine, Howard (nephew), Bill, Kikve (mother), John, Mary (John's wife) holding Harriet. Family detained at Minidoka Relocation Center in Idaho in 1942. The Cadet Nurse Corps provided Hideko and Geradine a way "out" and an opportunity to attend the Kahler School of Nursing in Rochester, Minnesota. Bill was a medical student and intern at the University of Michigan on the outbreak of World War II.

children. Theirs was a determination and endurance born, I would say, of an uncommon spirit.[8]

The Oriental Exclusion Act of 1924 abruptly stopped the flow of immigrants from Asia into the United States. The Japanese government was shocked. Ministers, teachers, treaty merchants, and students were allowed only temporary admittance. Those promoting the Act said that the language barrier would always be a problem.[9] Japan had agreed to American demands to restrict immigration, but to have their citizens barred from the United States was a blow to Japanese national pride.[10]

The Issei living in America could not become citizens. Anti-Japanese land legislation prohibited persons of Japanese ancestry from owning land in California and other western states. Their fellow countrymen could not enter the United States as immigrants. Most lacked money to go back to Japan. Their only hope rested in their American-born children, the "Nisei."[11] When the Issei generation acquired enough assets to purchase property, they bought property in the name of their citizen children.

The Japanese women who joined new and sometimes strange husbands in an unfamiliar country brought a sense of uplift to the Issei life in America. Two Nisei women, Miyeko "Mickie" Hayano Hara and Teruko "Teddy" Wada Tanaka, shared stories about their Japanese mothers who were well educated and encouraged their children in their school work while instilling an appreciation for their native Japanese language and cultural arts. They took on the responsibilities of maintaining a home as well as contributing to the family's enterprise of farming during those hard years of the Great Depression.

References and Notes

[1] Daisuke Kitagawa, *Issei and Nisei the Internment Years*, (New York: The Seabury Press, 1967):10.

[2] Jerry Stanley, *A True Story of Japanese Internment*, (New York: Delacorte Press, 1994):2.

[3] Linda Perrin, *Coming to America: Immigrants from the Far East*, (New York: Delacorte Press, 1980):69-70.

[4] Ibid, 73.

[5] Yancey, Diane, *Life in Japanese American Internment Camp*, (San Diego, California: Lucent Books, 1988):16-17.

[6] Ibid, 16.

[7] Ibid, 18.

[8] Yoshiko Uchida, *Desert Exile: The Uprooting of a Japanese American Family*, (Seattle: University of Washington Press, 1982):5-6.

[9] Kitagawa, 8.

[10] Perrin, 81.

[11] Bill Hosokawa, *Nisei The Quiet Americans: The Story of a People*, (New York: William Morrow and Company, Inc., 1969):123-8.

Teruko "Teddy" Wada Tanaka

*In Japan, mother had lived the life of a wealthy family with
lots of servants at her beck and call. She was aghast at the
primitive abode she found in the States. Pioneering was not
to her liking—she had never started a fire or even boiled
water.*

TERUKO "TEDDY" WADA TANAKA'S parents came to the United States
from Japan in the early 1900s. Kango Wada finished his high school
education in Japan and worked in banking before immigrating. He
landed in Seattle, Washington, and worked as a house boy while learning the English language. Kango worked on the railroads in the West
and then he decided to become a farmer leasing land in the Yakima
Valley in Oregon. Buying land was not allowed in California if one was
not a United States citizen, and Asian immigrants were not permitted
citizenship by naturalization at that time.

In the late 1920s, Kango heard of the Reclamation Project in
Eastern Oregon, so with two friends, he purchased a section of sage-
brush land that they cleared by hand and started to farm. When Mr.
Wada was 30 years old, he returned to Japan to marry Teddy's mother,
Nobue, whom he had known in his youth. "In Japan, Mother had lived
the life of a wealthy family with lots of servants at her beck and call,"
Teddy said. "She was aghast at the primitive abode she found in the
States." Pioneering was not to her liking; she had never started a fire or
even boiled water. She credited her evolution into becoming a hardworking mother of eight children to the patience of Teddy's father, who
taught her the essentials of everyday living.

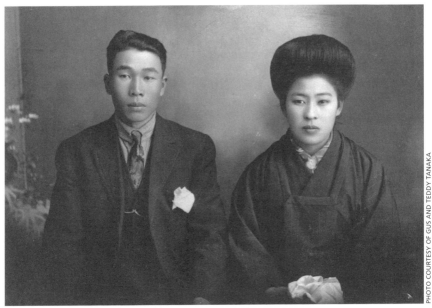

Kango and Nobue Wada. Wedding portrait, 1915.

Teddy remembers having great times as a child making huge bon-fires and eating charred potatoes. This was the beginning of the Great Depression, and it was a hand-to-mouth existence. Even though the Wada family was poor, education was of prime importance, and the Wada children walked to catch a bus that took them ten miles to school.

Teddy and her brothers and sisters grew up in an area where there were few Japanese, and they knew no discrimination. The highlight of their week was going into town to attend the Methodist Church. Even though Teddy's mother never learned to speak English well, she enjoyed the atmosphere of the church and the friendship. Eventually, through the work of Mr. Wada as a primary mover, a Japanese Methodist Church was established in Ontario, Oregon, with a Japanese and English speaking minister. Kango loved art, befriended starving artists, and became a master of Japanese calligraphy.

Teddy graduated from high school in 1940. Since her only hope for higher education was going to a large city and finding work to finance

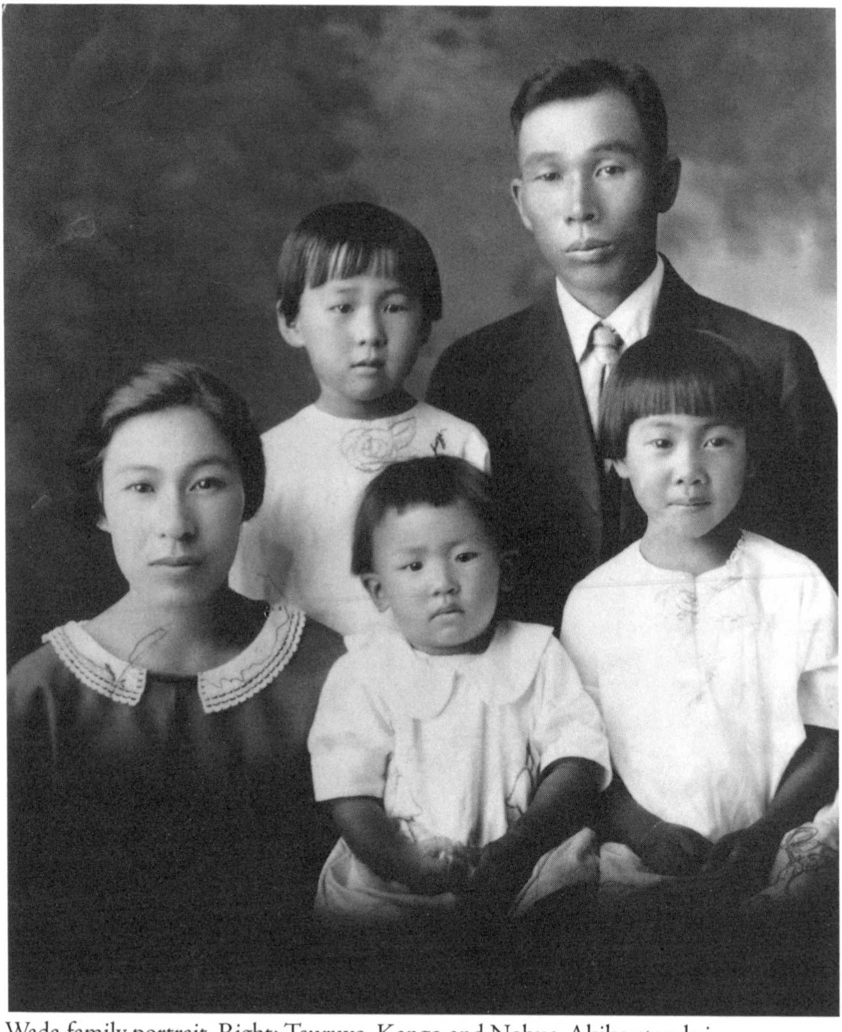
PHOTO COURTESY OF GUS AND TEDDY TANAKA

Wada family portrait. Right: Tsuruyo, Kango and Nobue. Akiko stands in rear between parents, Teruko, front center. Circa 1925.

her schooling, she traveled to Los Angeles, California. She joined her sister, who was attending a clothing design school while working as a maid part time. Following her sister's path, Teddy found housework, established residency, and enrolled in a pre-nursing program in Los Angeles. At that time, tuition was free, and she also worked part time in the library to buy books and supplies.

The Japanese attack on Pearl Harbor changed the lives of everyone in the entire nation, but it affected Japanese Americans living on the Pacific Coast, aliens and citizens alike, in unique ways. In March 1942, the Wartime Relocation Order on the West Coast gave Teddy a choice of either returning to her parents' home in eastern Oregon, or being evacuated. The Tanaka sisters were fortunate that their parents' home was just outside the military zone. Once home, the sisters were determined to find a way to continue their education and worked on the farm for one growing season. Their father was able to pay them enough wages for a year's tuition.

Teddy's goal was to become a nurse, which appealed to her desire to work with people and to "get ahead." Her mother was not happy with her choice of careers since nurses were classed as menial laborers in Japan. When she convinced her mother that nursing in the United States was a noble profession, she sought schools with her parents' blessings. She sent letters to schools of nursing throughout the Midwest and all the way to New York. Several schools responded negatively, giving reasons such as fear for Teddy's race not fitting in with the wartime efforts. St. Mary's Hospital School of Nursing in Rochester, Minnesota, an affiliate of the Mayo Clinic, was the first to offer an application. Teddy applied and was accepted in the June 1943 class.

Now Teddy had to find a way to get to Rochester. In January 1942, she took a bus to Denver, where she had a friend. She found another house maid job and earned enough money to buy a train ticket to Rochester. St. Mary's Hospital nuns, who ran the institution, did their utmost to make the Japanese American students feel a part of the community. During her years there, she never felt prejudice. In retrospect, Teddy said, "It was amazing since my classmates were all Midwestern girls who had no previous contact with Orientals as peers. This was a happy time—working hard, making friends, and realizing that together we were getting a nursing education in a school of nursing regarded as one of the best at that time."

The nuns knew Teddy had no money to pay for her second and third year tuition, so they worked out a plan for her to pay them back

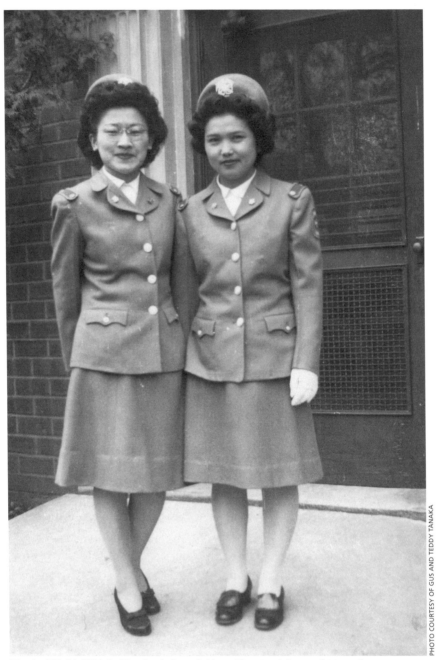

Teruko "Teddy" Wada Tanaka, left, and Alyce Shimizu Matsuuchi in cadet nurse uniform, 1945.

by working extra hours. Fortunately, the U.S. Cadet Nurse Corps was instituted at St. Mary's. Teddy was first in line to enlist, since her board and room, tuition, books, uniforms, and a stipend would be provided. In addition, it was great to know that as a cadet she would be doing her part in the war effort.

After graduation Teddy and her roommate, another Nisei, decided to go to New York City. Thanks to a scholarship Teddy received from St. Mary's, she attended Columbia University and earned a bachelor's degree in Oncology Nursing. She was working on her master's degree when she met and married Dr. Gus Tanaka, a resident in general surgery. This put an end to Teddy's nursing career. The Tanakas quickly started their family and were blessed with three children in three years. Teddy said, "I wouldn't say we were in a rush, but we were already 30 years old when we tied the knot."

Gus finished his residency in 1958, and the family decided to move back home to Ontario, Oregon, where Gus' father had established a general practice after the war. From that point on, Teddy assisted her husband in his practice. The couple retired in 1993 and now spends time enjoying their family, including five grandchildren, and traveling. Teddy has come a long way from humble beginnings, thanks in part to the Cadet Nurse Corps, and she gives thanks to the generosity of her wonderful nation.

Miyeko "Mickey" Hayano Hara

There were no divorcees among the picture brides.

MIYEKO "MICKEY" HAYANO HARA grew up in the Platte River Valley
in western Nebraska. Her father, Jusuke Hayano, was born in 1883 in
Fukushima-ken, Japan. At 22 years of age he immigrated to Hawaii
and worked in a sugar factory. In 1906, along with 18 friends, he went
to Nebraska and worked on the railroads. A couple of years later he
began farming in the Platte River Valley. Once established in farming in
Nebraska, Jusuke was ready for a family and sent for a Japanese bride.
Mickey's mother, Sumino, received her early education in Fukushima-
ken and worked as a governess. At age 26, the time was right for
Sumino, and a marriage was arranged by the families in Japan. Sumino
and Jusuke exchanged pictures and agreed to marry.

In 1920, along with other picture brides, Sumino boarded a steamship bound for Seattle, Washington. On board ship, the brides, holding
pictures of their future husbands, took part in a wedding ceremony.
Jusuke met his bride in Seattle, and they were married in a civil ceremony before traveling by train to Nebraska. Mickey later reflected,
"There were no divorcees among the picture brides. My parents' culture
taught them to accept *gaman*, which means to persevere and tough it
out, although there is no equivalent in the English language to describe
the depth of feeling."

Along with seven children, Sumino raised a garden and chickens.
She milked cows, fed the pigs, and enjoyed cooking, canning, sewing,
quilting, and crocheting. Mickey was the third child in her family and
grew up in rural America, much like other farm children during the
Great Depression. She rose early to do her assigned chores before

walking 5 miles each day to school in Henry, Nebraska. Along the way she and her siblings joined other children of German Russian immigrant families. Mickey said that their family always spoke Japanese at home; English was their second language. The family subscribed to many periodicals and newspapers, and Jusuke learned to read English.

The Hayano children helped in the field work of raising sugar beets, corn, beans, hay, and potatoes as well as tomatoes and peas which were sold to a cannery. They milked cows, fed pigs, and pumped water by hand for the work horses. In the summer when the farm work subsided a bit, the Hayano children attended a Japanese camp in Scottsbluff, Nebraska, conducted by university students from Japan. Mickey studied the Japanese language and learned a Japanese dance called *odori* wearing colorful Japanese kimonos. Mickey's knowledge of the Japanese language proved useful in writing to her mother while a student nurse away from home.

Mickey was 17 when Pearl Harbor was bombed. The mayor of Henry visited the family and told them that there would be no trouble. All they had to do was to turn in their guns, cameras, and short-wave radios. Mickey said that there were incidences of Caucasian children stopping by to walk with Japanese American friends to school to make sure there was no reprisal.

Upon graduation from high school, Mickey received a scholarship to the University of Nebraska, but her family could not afford to pay the other expenses. Mickey had worked on the farm for one year and planned to join the Women's Army Corps. Then she learned about the U.S. Cadet Nurse Corps from a friend. Formation of the Corps in mid-1943 became the answer for an acute shortage of nurses. Increasing the number of student nurses who gave service while they learned ultimately added to the supply of graduate nurses and greatly supplemented the total nurse power of the nation. In the process student nurses were given the satisfaction of making a contribution to the war effort.[1]

Any young woman who could meet the admission requirements of an approved school of nursing participating in the federal program was eligible to join the U.S. Cadet Nurse Corps. Out of Government funds, the school transmitted to her a complete scholarship and a monthly stipend as her personal allowance. In return the Cadets agreed to remain in essential nursing service, military or civilian, for the duration of the war. The cadet also received a complete outdoor uniform.[2]

Mickey discovered that a small Catholic school of nursing in Colorado Springs, Colorado was accepting Nisei students. She completed the necessary forms and her application to the Seton School of Nursing was approved. Fifteen Japanese American students were admitted to Seton between 1943 and 1945. The nuns were strict, and the students received a good nursing education. The nuns also required their cadets to learn how to march. Drill sergeants were called out from Fort Carson to instruct the cadets. The cadets wore white blouses and navy pants and made a good presentation when a commanding officer reviewed them.

When Mickey completed her nursing education, she had no problem in finding a nursing position. This also enabled her to assist a younger sister in attending college. After many years of active nursing service in the Nebraska community, Mickey now volunteers as a nurse and writes and gives presentations regarding the history of the Japanese in Nebraska.

Notes

[1] United States Federal Security Agency. (1950). *The U.S. Cadet Nurse Corps 1943-1948*. (Public Health Service Publication No. 38) (Washington, D.C.: Government Printing Office):18-19.

[2] Ibid, 18-19.

2 Growing Up American: The Nisei

T HE NISEI GROWING UP in America had both Japanese and American ancestry. Their parents, the Issei, were Japanese citizens who had immigrated to America to better their lives. Nisei (pronounced *nee say*) children were the first generation to be born in America and were automatically citizens according to law. Before 1924, Nisei had dual citizenship with Japan because of their ancestry. After 1924, Issei parents had to register their children in Japan if they desired dual citizenship. Most parents did not make this effort, although Issei retained strong ties to Japan and exposed their children to its traditions. The Issei spoke Japanese, often lived in Japanese communities, and kept their Japanese manners and customs. Like all traditional Japanese, they demanded strict obedience from their children and expected them to conform to authority and to community standards. They admonished their children not to bring disgrace upon their family or community and expected them to do their best in every undertaking.[1]

The majority of the Issei's children, the Nisei, were born between 1910 and 1940. Both boys and girls began at an early age to help with the family's enterprise, usually a small business or farm. The Nisei growing up in rural America resembled other American farm children during the Great Depression; it was a time when children did chores and worked on the farms and ranches, contributing to their family's welfare. Nisei growing up in urban areas helped in their family's small businesses, and making do was a way of life. There was little money, but those years were filled with warmth and love for many.

The Nisei integrated both the Japanese customs of their parents and the ways of their American friends and classmates. Most grew up speaking Japanese with their parents and English with their friends and teachers. A large segment of the Nisei attended Japanese language school, often held after public school hours, making for a long day of education. The programs were diverse but typically embodied and taught respect for parents and elders, self-reliance, obligation, hard work, and other Japanese virtues. The language schools provided a stage for Japanese folklore, plays, songs, and dances emphasizing Japanese ethics that in many instances parallel the "Puritan work ethic."[2]

Many Issei were Buddhist, but most Nisei were Christian. Parents and children together enjoyed celebrating the New Year with traditional foods and by visiting other Japanese families. They also celebrated Thanksgiving and Christmas. The girls learned to knit, sew, and embroider, and some took lessons in Japanese folk dancing. The boys played baseball and football and turned on the radio for *Gangbusters*. The adolescent Nisei listened to the *Hit Parade* and danced to the big bands of the time.[3]

A prevailing widespread belief in the Japanese community was that a person of a minority race had to have much higher qualification than a Caucasian to get a job. Hence the Nisei tended to concentrate their energies on school work. The experience of discipline within their own homes was a factor in the formation of study practices that contributed to the success of the college bound Japanese American student.[4]

The Nisei thought of themselves as Americans, but there was discrimination when it came to getting good jobs. In 1930 the Nisei formed the Japanese American Citizen League (JACL), which was influential in Washington, Oregon, and California where 95 percent of Japanese Americans lived. The purpose of the JACL was to fight discrimination against the Japanese and to demonstrate their loyalty.[5]

A Nisei, Mike Masaoka, wrote the JACL's creed sometime in 1940, conveying the super-Americanism expressed by many of the members:

I am proud that I am an American citizen of Japanese ancestry, for my very background makes me appreciate more fully the wonderful advantages of this nation. I believe in her institutions, ideals and tradition: I glory in her heritage; I boast of her history; I trust in her future.[6]

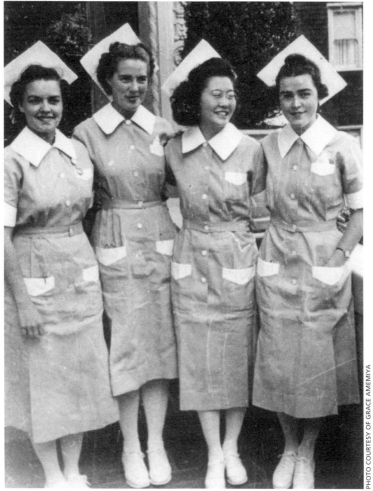

Grace Obata (second from right), student nurse at the University of California School of Nursing, completed one semester before evacuation (Fall 1941).

PHOTO COURTESY OF GRACE AMEMIYA

The Issei were strict and not inclined to open displays toward their children. However, the Nisei were aware of their parents' concern for them and the family. The family's strength and responsibility helped sustain them through economic hardship and discrimination. Together they faced the anti-Japanese movement of the 1920s and the Great Depression of the 1930s.

Like their American peers, the Nisei women remember when every able-bodied man, woman, and child worked at something to bring in a dollar here and there. "Make it over, wear it out, make it do, or do without," was the cliché for those hard economic times. Some schools and banks promoted savings programs to teach children the virtues of thrift. For Margaret Baba Yasuda, her small savings would buy her a ticket to freedom. Like other Nisei, Ida Sakohira Kawaguchi recalls those times and speaks of courage, strength, and the family love that saw her through.

References and Notes

[1] Diane Yancey, *Life in Japanese Internment Camp*, (San Diego, California: Lucent Books, 1988):19.

[2] Report of the Commission on Wartime Relocation and Internment of Civilians, *Personal Justice Denied* (Washington, D.C., Government Printing Office, 1962):39. The commission's report included hearings and archival research and took testimony from more than 750 witnesses. Between July 1961 and December 1982, the Commission staff collected and reviewed materials from government and university archives, read as well as analyzed the relevant historical writing.

[3] Valerie Matsumoto, "Japanese American Women During World War II," *Frontiers* 8, no. 1 (1949)7.

[4] Robert W. O'Brien, *The College Nisei*, (Palo Alto, California: Pacific Books, 1994):8.

[5] Jerry Stanley. *A True Story of Japanese Internment*, (New York: Crown Publishers, 1994):2.

[6] Yancey, 22.

Margaret Baba Yasuda

The children of immigrant families were expected to work when not in school. Immigrant children should persevere and not complain.

IN 1938 MARGARET BABA was 14 years of age. She had grown up in Seattle, Washington, and now it was time to join her sister and her sister's friend for summer work. A ferry cruising toward Vashon Island took them to their destination, where they would spend the summer picking berries. Thinking this would be a leisurely vacation, Margaret was soon jolted from her dream. The next day found her toiling under the blistering sun on a strawberry farm. In the beginning Margaret bent over the low plants, admiring the huge luscious strawberries and eating a few. But the berries got smaller and smaller while the strawberry field seemed to grow larger and larger, stretching forever with the end of the field farther and farther away.

Soon Margaret found she could no longer bend over the plants. She squatted and scooted, and her pants became crusted with mashed berries and dirt. Her knees became as stiff as a telephone pole and she could hardly walk. The farmer's wife cooked the meals and made lunches for the pickers. Sometimes the farmer brought the pickers a cup of ice cold water. What a treat!

When the strawberries shriveled up the girls headed for the loganberry fields. This was better since they could pick the berries standing up. However, Margaret's knees swelled and walking became excruciating. Immigrant children were expected to work when not in school. Margaret remembered the motto "Immigrant children should persevere and not complain." Margaret was determined to finish the summer in the berry fields. Limping and groaning, somehow she made it through that long hot summer. Finally the girls were home.

Margaret's mother took one look at her child's frail body and swollen knee joints and took her to the doctor. She was diagnosed with arthritis in both knees, a disease that would continue to plague her throughout her life. Through the experience Margaret began to appreciate and admire the doctors and nurses who ministered to her. By the time she graduated from high school, Margaret knew that nursing was for her.

When the war broke out, those of Japanese ancestry, including Margaret and her family, were first interned at the Puyallup Assembly Center in Washington. They were surrounded by barbed wire fences and security guards. Margaret continued to hope that she could someday be a nurse but worried deep inside. How would she pay the tuition? Would they let her our of prison? How would she survive on her own? Could she leave her parents locked up in camp?

The situation in the assembly center was not good. Food was scarce. Would she and her family starve there? One day, they only had rice to eat. She put salt on her portion and swallowed hard. There was nothing else. Then the residents in Block 34 got food poisoning and 40 were hospitalized. Margaret wanted to get out of this "prison" and wrote to all former high school teachers asking for character reference letters.

After the move to the Minidoka Relocation Center in Idaho Margaret began writing letters to the State Boards of Nursing in many states asking for a list of schools of nursing. When she received the list of nursing schools, she diligently wrote each school requesting a brochure. She eliminated schools that refused to admit students of Japanese ancestry. After filling out endless numbers of applications, on March 18, 1943, Margaret received a letter of acceptance from the Seton School of Nursing in Colorado Springs, Colorado. The Catholic nuns who ran the school wrote that she could enroll in the July class.

On April 5 1943, Margaret received a special delivery letter releasing her from the Minidoka Relocation Center where she and her family

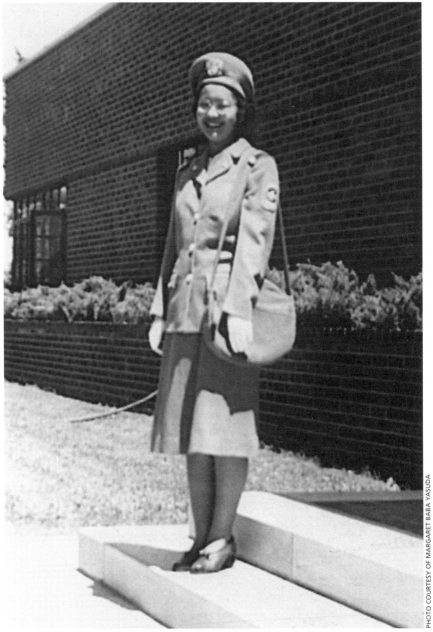

Cadet Nurse Margaret Baba, student nurse at Seton School of Nursing in Colorado Springs, Colorado, was inducted into the Corps on May 13, 1944.

were interned. Margaret was overjoyed. The tuition at the school was $214.50 for the three-year course with room, board, and laundry. As a student Margaret was informed that she would work in the hospital through her junior and senior years with no pay. Margaret wrote to the Washington Mutual Bank in Seattle and requested the $273.70 she had in her school savings account. The 5¢ a week that she saved all through her school days would pay her tuition and the train fare from Idaho to Colorado.

When the U.S. Cadet Nurse Corps became available in 1943, Margaret was inducted into the program. Now she would not have to worry about paying tuition or other expenses. She had jumped all the hurdles. Margaret was on her way to becoming a nurse. Margaret graduated from the Seton Hospital School of Nursing in 1946 and returned to Seattle, Washington where she began work on her bachelors degree at the University of Washington. On campus she met her future husband, Ted, a student in research library science. Margaret worked at the King County Health Department as a public health nurse for more than 20 years. The Yasudas raised three children and after 55 years of married life continue to enjoy life in Seattle along with their grandchildren.

Ida Sakohira Kawaguchi, Part 1

The timing of my high school graduation had an important meaning to me. I was in the last class to graduate before incarceration in the Gila River Relocation Center in Arizona. I was proud and happy to be chosen to start the graduation program with the invocation.

IDA SAKOHIRA's father, Kumataro Sakohira, settled in the fertile San Joaquin Valley and raised grapes in the small community of Fowler, California. The Sakohira family included six children: Elizabeth, Harry, Frank, Ruth, Tod, and Ida. Kumataro's first wife died of complications of childbirth when Ruth was born. He returned to Japan to find a wife and mother for his children. The second Mrs. Sakohira, Mitsuye Sakohira, after arriving in America often spoke of the difficulty of having to care for a ready-made family of four children. Todd and Ida were born of this marriage.

Ida's father rented a grape ranch in Fowler where Ida spent her childhood. Mitsuye would place baby Ida in a buggy and wheel her into the vineyards while she worked. Food and clothing for the family were purchased on credit and paid for when the grapes were harvested and sold. After many, many years of hard work, Kumataro managed to purchase his own grape ranch. The family lived in a small house on the property. There was a kitchen and three small rooms but no electricity or running water.

The boys helped run the ranch. The sisters were assigned domestic chores in the home. After school all the children helped with outside farm chores. They pumped water, filling buckets to carry to the watering trough for the horse as well as carrying water into the house for cooking and washing dishes. The children pumped water for the *furo*, which is a Japanese-style bath that is still a custom in Japan today. The tub was filled with water, then a fire was built under the tub to heat the water. The bath water was kept clean by washing and rinsing oneself outside the tub before jumping in to enjoy the luxury of relaxing in the deep, hot water. The children had a great time taking baths together.

The grapes had to be harvested before the rain. This was a crucial and busy time and extra help was hired. The family's livelihood depended on making the right decisions as to when to begin the harvest. There was a joint effort between family and hired help to get the grapes harvested before the rain. All worked long hours and looked forward to the last day of harvest when the parents would be relieved. Then the family celebrated with creamy and delicious homemade ice cream churned in an old-fashioned ice cream maker. Ida's father enjoyed his home-brewed beer, which he continued to make after prohibition. The beer was secretly stored in the bottom of the well, accessible only by climbing down some steep steps. For a special visitor, Ida was chosen to bring up the beer, which she loved to do.

Summer in the San Joaquin Valley is hot, with temperatures soaring above 100 Fahrenheit. Pleasant childhood memories for Ida include swimming in the ditch alongside the property and in one area where there was a waterfall. Since the water was deep there, the children swam and dove into the swimming hole. When the Fowler High School built an outdoor swimming pool, the family went there, as it was bigger, safer, and much nicer.

Winters were cold with sometimes below-freezing weather. When the weather report predicted a frost, the farmers rushed to protect their crops by lighting smudge pots. The Sakohira family had a wood-burning stove in the kitchen for cooking that was also the sole source of heat. In the winter, the children dressed beside the warm stove. Ida loved rainy days because her father gave the children a ride home from school in the farm truck. Their mother had hot-baked cookies waiting for a special treat. Ida recalls that her mother was a great cook and learned to make tortillas from Mexican friends. She has pleasant memories of her mother rolling out tortillas and then cooking them on top of the stove.

Japanese parents sent their children to the Japanese school on Saturdays. Ida said that she never took those classes in reading and writing seriously. Before the summer break there was always a graduation program. All the students were required to participate in some way—performing a recitation, singing a Japanese song, or taking part in a Japanese dance. Japanese parents thought preserving their "roots" was important.

The Sakohira family life centered around the home for entertainment. Favorite radio programs were *Lone Ranger, Major Bowles' Amateur Hour, Fibber McGee and Molly, One Man's Family,* and *Little Orphan Annie.* Ida remembers walking a mile into town where the librarian helped the children select interesting books. Like many children growing up in the Great Depression, the Sakohira children had few toys and played games such as *Hide and Seek* and *Cops and Robbers.* They also played card games such as *Rummy* or *Twenty One.* Marbles occupied them for hours. Sports equipment included skates, balls and bicycles. Sometimes the family listened to records played on the hand-cranked Victrola, an early record player.

Ida's father had kidney disease. One winter he caught a cold and became seriously ill, and died. Also in her young life, Ida experienced the death of her stepbrother, who died as a result of an automobile accident. For Ida, attending a Buddhist funeral as a child was a frightening experience with the chanting, gongs, and incense burning.

Pearl Harbor uprooted the Sakohira family's rural life. The family lived beyond the prohibitive zone and was not sent to an assembly center, but it was required to observe curfew between 8 p.m. and 6 a.m. Signs were posted informing all those of Japanese ancestry that they would be relocated. The family made arrangements with a neighbor to care for their farm. During their incarceration they received no remuneration for the use of their farm.

June 1942 was a special time for Ida. "The timing of my high school graduation had importance to me," Ida remembered. "I was in the last class to graduate before incarceration in the Gila River Relocation Center in Arizona. I was proud and happy to be chosen to start the graduation program with the invocation."

It was a long, hot, and uncomfortable train ride to Gila River with armed guards and curtains drawn. Because of the intense heat and to prevent problems with dehydration, salt pills were passed out. When the evacuees finally reached their destination, they found a barren land surrounded by a barbed wire fence, watch towers, and armed sentries. The lack of privacy was disturbing. Later, the family purchased fabrics through the Montgomery Ward catalog and surrounded each bed with a curtain. Showers were taken in one large open room with no partitions. When the gong sounded at mealtime, the evacuees formed a line to the mess hall where they were served budget foods cafeteria style.

Living in close proximity to others, the Japanese American teenagers socialized easily. Movies were shown once a week at the outdoor theater, which had no seats. After dinner Ida and her family would head for the theater carrying their homemade folding chairs. Block dances were soon organized This was the era of big band music including *Benny Goodman, Tommy Dorsey, Glen Miller, Duke Ellington,* jazz, and jitterbug dancing. The young boys wore wide-legged trousers and were known as "zoot suiters." Sweaters. skirts, and brown and white saddle oxfords were popular with the girls. Protestant services were organized by Reverend Paul Osumi from Hawaii. The Japanese American teenagers thought their minister was "cool" and knew he understood them. He allowed social dancing in the barrack turned into a church.

When Ida heard that nurse aide classes were being offered at the camp hospital, she jumped at the chance to enroll. The hospital had an operating room and a delivery room with a bare minimum of equipment. Wards, double rooms, and a few single rooms for the patients were sparse. The hospital was staffed by evacuee surgeons, physicians, some student nurses, a few registered nurses, and nurse aides, who carried out the brunt of the ward work. Ida admired and looked up to the Japanese American registered nurses.

The nurse aides and orderlies were given the opportunity to observe childbirth and surgical procedures. Here they experienced life at an early age—death, the pain of labor and childbirth and the psychotic reaction of a patient after a mastectomy. The nurse aides were paid $16 a month, and the doctors were paid $19 a month. When Ida worked the swing or midnight shift, the hospital staff were picked up by the ambulance driver, as there was no transportation system in camp. Ida said that they were fortunate to have a professional cook at the hospital, and the nurse aides enjoyed eating there. Everything he cooked tasted good and was visually appealing, unlike the food served in the mess hall.

After a year of internment, there was an opportunity for residents to accept jobs outside of the camp. Ida heard about the U.S. Cadet Nurse Corps. She filled out an application form to clear her leave from the interment camp and also applied to several schools of nursing. She was elated when she received a letter of acceptance from St. Mary's School of Nursing in Rochester, Minnesota.

During this time the U.S. Army carried out a recruitment drive in the Gila River Camp. All draft able men were required to fill out a questionnaire and respond to questions regarding their loyalty to the United States. Prior to the questionnaire, physically fit draft-age Japanese American men were classified 4C, an enemy alien denied the opportunity to serve in the military, even though they were loyal Americans. There was much discussion among the men about the issue; some were bitter that they were incarcerated in camp, yet being asked to serve in the Army. Most answered "yes" to the loyalty questions. Those who answered "no" were considered a security risk and sent to citizen isolation camps.

The Japanese American men who volunteered for military intelligence shortened the war by two years, according to some historians, by intercepting secret messages, interrogating Japanese prisoners, and translating battle plan documents. Ida's future husband, Masaru, served with this unit. Ida's brothers, Frank and Todd, volunteered for the U.S. Army. Frank was sent to Harvard to teach Japanese reading and writing, and Todd was soon off to Camp Shelby, Mississippi, for basic training. Ida's brother, Harry, had volunteered early and was serving in the Army before evacuation. Ida remembers:

> The day I left camp was a sad one for me. This was the first time I would be away from my family for such a long period of time. When it was time to load the bus, I was in tears as I waved goodbye to my family. I was happy that there were some familiar faces on the bus to keep me company. I was scared as this was the first time I would be on my own.

3 The Shock of War

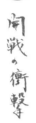

THE BOMBING OF PEARL HARBOR on December 7, 1941 changed the lives of everyone in our country, but for the Japanese American citizens and aliens living in the declared military zone, a profound disruption took over their peaceful lives. Panic swept the West Coast during the days following Pearl Harbor. A Japanese invasion seemed imminent. Rumors and alarms were rampant; cities were blacked out. A curfew required persons of Japanese ancestry to be in their homes between 8 p.m. and 6 a.m.[1]

Fear of the Japanese in America persisted despite the fact that no evidence of subversive activity was found among those with Japanese ancestry. On February 19, 1942, President Frankllin Roosevelt signed Executive Order 9066, authorizing the War Department to exclude from designated military areas all those considered a threat to national security. Some 110,000 people with Japanese ancestry, more than 60 percent of them citizens and 40,000 of them children, would be evacuated.[2]

One Japanese American nurse wrote that she was 18 years old and a senior in high school when she learned about the evacuation. She said that this was a time of much confusion and anxiety. She added that she had blocked these events out of her mind and to this day could not remember the details.[3]

On February 23, 1942, an enemy submarine shelled Goleta, California, near Santa Barbara; it was a timely act from the standpoint of the exclusionists. General John L. DeWitt, commanding officer of the Army Western Defense Command, lost no time in designating the western half of the three Pacific Coast states and the southern third of Arizona as Military Area No.1. General DeWitt stipulated that all persons of Japanese descent would be removed from this area. Vilolating an order was a federal offense. Prior to March 27, 1942, the Wartime Civil Control Administration (WCCA) permitted voluntary movement out of the designated war zone. After this date futher voluntary migration of citizens with Japanese ancestry was forbiden. Life was too uncertain for Japanese families, and few could take advantage of this opportunity anyway. Most families had no alternative but to stay and let the government take action.[4] The War Relocation Authority was created to assist persons evacuated by the military. Milton S. Eisenhower, brother of General Dwight D. Eisenhower, was named the first director.[5]

Could Nisei faith in the ideals and values of the American culture be rekindled? Early in May 1942, California Governor Culbert Olson wrote a letter to President Roosevelt relaying the concern of the Western College Association regarding the evacuation of loyal Japanese American students. The Governor said that such a move would be injurious not only to the students, but also to the nation since well-trained leadership for such persons would be needed during and after the war.[6] President Roosevelt promptly replied and wrote as follows:

I am deeply concerned that the American-born Japanese college students shall be impressed with the ability of the American people to distinguish between enemy aliens and staunch supporters of the American system who happen to have Japanese ancestry.[7]

As graduate nurses joined the military, our country faced the most critical nurse shortage in history. Retired nurses were pressed into military service. The Red Cross began training thousands of nurses' aides to take over some of the basic nursing tasks. One plan was to recruit more young women into nursing schools. Nurse leader Isabel Stewart pointed out that most of the students' education was in the hospital providing care so they were an obvious source of nursing service needed in civilian and military hospitals. In fact, during this time, student nurses provided the largest percentage of nursing service in hospitals that were affiliated with nursing schools.[8]

May Kurose Joichi, a Nisei student nurse at the Washington University School of Nursing, was helping to compensate for the loss of registered nurses to military service before the evacuation. Now she had to leave her school and nursing assignments and look for ways to continue her nursing education. The Seattle Chapter of the Japanese American Citizens League (JACL) made every effort to cooperate with the government to facilitate early evacuation measures. May benefited from their assistance.

After Sumiko "Sammie" Itoi Brinsfield received her high school diploma at the Minidoka Relocation High School, she signed up for a nurse aide course. These skills helped her find a job from which she learned about the U.S. Cadet Nurse Corps.

References and Notes

[1] Report of the Commission on Wartime Relocation and Internment of Civilians, *Personal Justice Denied*, (Washington, D.C.: Government Printing Office, 1982):101.

[2] Robert James Maddox, *The United States and World War II*, (Boulder, Colorado: Westview Press, 1992):97-8.

[3] Anonymous, correspondence to author, Nisei Cadet Nurse Project, (Boulder, Colorado: 6 January 2001).

[4] Report, 101-3.

[5] Dillon S. Myer, *Uprooted Americans: The Japanese Americans and the War Relocation Authority during World War II*, (Tucson, Arizona: The University of Arizona Press, 1971):xxiv.

[6] Bill Hosokawa, *Nisei: the Quiet Americans: The Story of a People*, (New York: William Morrow and Company, Inc., 1969):351-2

[7] Ibid.

[8] Thelma M. Robinson and Paulie Perry, *Cadet Nurse Stories: The Call For and Response of Women During World War II*, (Indianapolis, Indiana: Center Nursing Press, 2001):4.

May Kurose Joichi

*Having lived a sheltered life, I was fearful about my future
in a strange city far away. I left Seattle on the day the first
curfew took effect to finish my education in Chicago.*

MAY KUROSE JOICHI'S decision to become a nurse was made at a
young age. She was eight years old when both parents were hospitalized in Seattle, Washington. While visiting them in the hospital, she
observed nurses in white starched uniforms and caps caring for her
parents. She decided she wanted to be a nurse so she could help others.

The Kurose family lived in a Japanese community and went to public
schools. After school May attended Japanese language school taught
by her mother. The family attended the Japanese Baptist Church and
other religious groups such as the Baptist Young Peoples' Union and
World Wide Guild. They also participated in the Japanese American
sports league by playing basketball and baseball.

When the war broke out, the Kuroses learned about curfew, the
assembly centers, and relocation centers from the JACL. However, they
weren't told when all of this would take effect. May, now 20 years old,
was enrolled in the University of Washington School of Nursing and
had been accepted into the sorority Alpha Tau Delta.

Before curfew in Seattle took effect, May's parents decided that
she should finish her schooling in Chicago. Through the help of the
JACL, she received her leave permit and a sponsorship from the Baptist
Missionary School in Chicago. "Having lived a sheltered life, I was
fearful about my future in a strange city far away," May said. "I left
Seattle on the day the first curfew took effect to finish my education in
Chicago. I was met at the Chicago Union Station by three wonderful

students of the Baptist Missionary School. They were understanding and kind, and I soon found a job as a nurse aide at the Chicago Children's Memorial Hospital."

May sent many letters of application to schools of nursing in Iowa, Minnesota, Michigan, and Illinois but received no answer. During this time she had difficulty finding an apartment to rent because of her Japanese ancestry. Her Nisei friend and she decided to say they were Koreans, and they soon found lodging.

May heard about the Mercy Hospital School of Nursing, which was affiliated with St. Xavier College in Chicago. She applied and was interviewed by Sister Mary Therese, R.S.M., and May found her to be the most wonderful, progressive, and loving individual she had ever met. Sister Mary Therese accepted May's application and told her that if she did well, more Japanese American students would be admitted. Sure enough, at least four more students were accepted in classes to follow.

Opportunity soon rang for May to become a member of the U.S. Cadet Nurse Corps. "The general public had been good to me, and I felt no animosity towards joining a United States uniformed service even though my parents were interned at the Minidoka Relocation Center," May recollected about her decision to join.

May visited her parents in camp wearing her cadet nurse uniform. She was surprised when guards flirted with her. She wanted to spend her senior cadet nurse experience at a veterans hospital but was told that this might not be a good idea due to the returning South Pacific soldiers. May specialized in the operating room instead. After graduation she pursued further training and received certification in Operating Room Technique and Supervision at Yale University School of Nursing. May retired in June, 1985 after 35 years of teaching students operating room technique and supervising departments of surgery.

In retrospect, May said, "Since my enrollment at the St. Xavier College School of Nursing and throughout my career as an employee of many hospitals, I have not experienced discrimination due to my ancestry. People of all races have been good to me. As far as joining the Cadet Nurse Corps, I was glad to be part of the United States uniformed services during World War II."

Sumiko "Sammie" Itoi Brinsfield

How could anyone think that our quiet, hardworking
father would have any furtive motives?

Sumiko "Sammie" Itoi Brinsfield's mother, Benke Nigikee
Nagakima, was the daughter of a Congregational minister in Japan who
brought his family of two daughters and two sons to the United States.
At age 16 Benke married Seizo Itoi, who had studied law in Japan
before departing for the United States to seek a different life. In Seattle,
Seizo operated a hotel with rooms and a large dormitory mainly for
men who were laborers, widowers, and retirees. Benke enjoyed writing
poetry with other like-minded friends, and they held monthly gather-
ings at each other's homes. She wrote regular articles about Japanese
women that were published in newspapers and magazines in Japan.

Sammie had an older sister, Monica, and a brother. Another brother,
Kenje, died from cholera when the family was traveling on a steamship
to Japan to visit grandparents. The Itoi children grew up in the Japanese
community and attended public schools. The family were members
of the Japanese Methodist Church. Sammie belonged to a choir and
enjoyed singing in Handel's "Messiah." Other fond memories include
the annual church bazaars with ethnic foods, games, and booths set up
with beautiful Japanese handcrafted items.

On December 7, 1941, the Itoi family went to church as usual
and were greeted by anxious friends who told them that Japanese
planes had bombed Pearl Harbor. A curfew had been ordered for the
Japanese community, and every night they were to be in their homes
by 8 p.m. Several days later FBI agents were incarcerating men, and
agents appeared on their doorstep. Sammie thought, "How could

anyone think that our quiet, hardworking father would have any furtive motives?"

Sammie's parents taught their children to be conscientious American citizens. Her older brother, a pre-med student, was attending the University of Washington at the outbreak of World War II. He had applied to medical schools but was not accepted because of his race. Her older sister had been attending secretarial school, but she contracted tuberculosis and was in a sanitarium for cure.

Sammie was a junior at Franklin High School and recalls the Spanish language class teacher asking the Nisei students to step outside the classroom. She learned later that the principal had instructed the teachers to speak to the rest of the student body and remind them that Nisei students were Americans and were not responsible for what happened at Pearl Harbor. Everything went well, and Sammie does not remember any harassment. She is grateful for the principal's sensitivity.

One evening the family had run out of toilet paper, and since Sammie was female and the youngest member in the family—a threat to no one—she volunteered to run down the block to a neighbor's house to borrow the much-needed item. This took place after the 8 p.m. curfew, and Sammie accomplished the mission without a hitch. She felt like a heroine in a movie. A few weeks later the family was escorted by armed military guards to the Puyallup Assembly Center in Washington. Later they were transferred by bus and train to the Minidoka Relocation Center in Twin Falls, Idaho. The soldiers, mostly young men with rifles, stood guard around them.

Sammie remembers the desert land with cacti scattered across the horizon and the dust storms. Sand blew through the cracks into the room the family shared. They hung blankets across one corner to give privacy while dressing. Residents signed up to fill positions as cooks, policemen, teachers, doctors, and nurses, and the internment camp became self-sufficient.

Makeshift classrooms were set up for elementary and high school children. Their Nisei chemistry teacher had a single Bunsen burner to demonstrate the reaction of chemicals. After Sammie received her

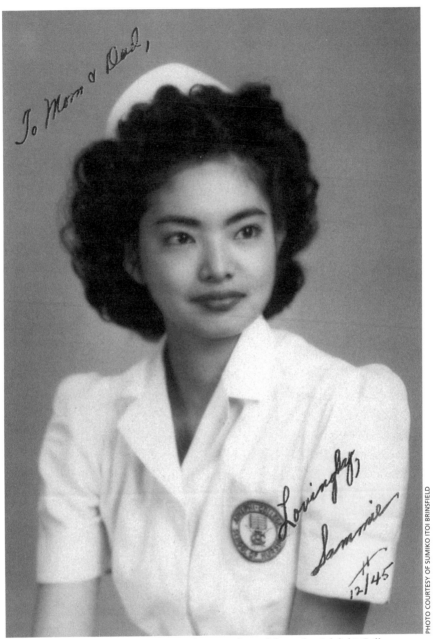

To Mom & Dad,

Lovingly,
Sammie
12/45

Sumiko (Sammie) Itoi, in hospital uniform, graduated from the Adelphi College School of Nursing in New York in 1946.

high school diploma, there was a need for nurse aides and she signed up. Months later the evacuees were given permission to leave as long as they agreed not to go back to the Pacific Coast. Sammie gladly took the monetary compensation of $25 to cover bus and train fare to the Midwest. Sammie said, "I'm sure my parents felt some foreboding to see their young daughter going out into the unknown where feelings towards the 'enemy' were at an all-time high."

Sammie went to Indianapolis, Indiana, and lived with a minister and his wife. She used her nurse aide skills to find a job and learned about the U.S. Cadet Nurse Corps. She applied to the Adelphi College School of Nursing located in Garden City, Long Island, New York, and was accepted, making her eligible for induction into the Corps.

Sammie's classmates at Adelphi College came from all walks of life, with all the major religions represented. First Lady Eleanor Roosevelt visited the campus to encourage and inspire the cadets. Being in the Cadet Nurse Corps gave young women discipline, pride, and a sense of purpose. Sammie said, "I was aware that my classmates were more jovial and carefree than I. My thoughts were always with my parents interned in camp. My cadet nurse stipend of $20 a month made it possible to send food and clothing to them from time to time. Being on my own for the first time and so far from my family, I learned to become independent and self-sufficient."

Sammie was grateful to be able to pursue her interest in nursing and to prove her loyalty to the United States. She had planned to join the Army, but World War II had ended when she graduated, and the large number of military nurses was no longer needed. She married a non-Japanese who also grew up in Seattle. The Brinsfields have been married for more than 50 years.

Sammie reflects on their bond:

My parents gave us their blessing. They said that my husband was just like a Nisei. We have two handsome sons. My life has been interesting in sharing it with my husband, whose career was an attorney and later on as Chief Executive Officer of four stock exchange companies. My husband was diagnosed with Parkinson's Disease in 1980. My training as a nurse has served me well, thanks to the U.S. Cadet Nurse Corps.

4 The Uprooting

追
い
五
了

A six-year-old Nisei boy said to a Caucasian, a university professor who had come down to help evacuees with their luggage, "Are you going to Puyallup (Assembly Center) with us?"

"No, sonny," said the white man. "I can't go with you."

"Gee," was the answer. "Ain't you sorry you ain't Japanese!"

To the children the excitement of skipping school, packing, getting up early, taking the big bus—most of them had never traveled before in their lives—was a picnic. Next day these same school children were inside the fence at Puyallup Assembly Center, hanging on the wire looking out at white children riding their bicycles or on roller skates—there was nothing to do inside—no place to go—the picnic was over.[1]

ON MARCH 31, 1942, the evacuation began. Through August 7, 1942, groups of around 500 with Japanese ancestry were escorted by the army from their homes to assembly centers or to a relocation center as directed by one of the 108 "Civilian Exclusion Orders."[2]

The task of evacuating families was formidable. The Japanese were required to report and register to "civil control stations" that were located in all centers of the Japanese population. Each member of an evacuation family was given the same identification number. Evacuees

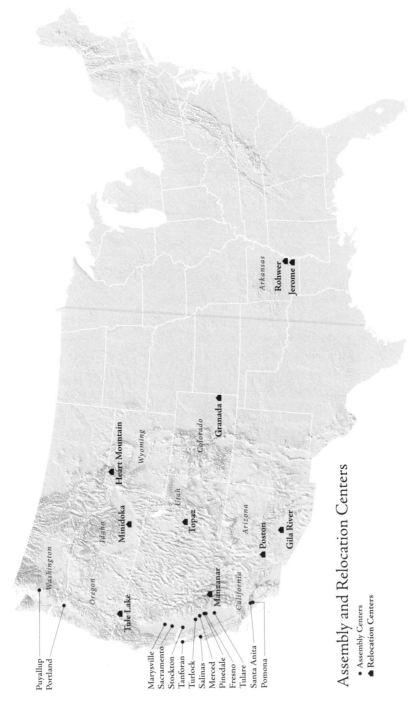

Assembly and Relocation Centers

- Assembly Centers
- ▲ Relocation Centers

Arkansas

Rohwer ▲
Jerome ▲

Granada ▲

Colorado

Wyoming

Heart Mountain ▲

Utah

Idaho

Minidoka ▲

Topaz ▲

Arizona

Poston ▲

Gila River ▲

Washington

Oregon

Tule Lake ▲

Manzanar ▲

California

Puyallup
Portland

Marysville
Sacramento
Stockton
Tanforan
Turlock
Salinas
Merced
Pinedale
Fresno
Tulare
Santa Anita
Pomona

were then told to wind up affairs, store or sell their possessions, close businesses and homes, and report to a designated assembly point at a specific time. On departure day they were told to bring only what they could carry and to include the following items: bedding and linens, toilet articles, extra clothing, forks, spoons, plates, bowls and cups for each member of the family. Essential personal items that would be needed should be brought, but no pets of any kind would be permitted.[3]

About 92,000 people with Japanese ancestry were evacuated to assembly centers, where they remained for an average of about 100 days. All fourteen assembly centers were in California, except for Puyallup in Washington and Portland in Oregon. On departure day the evacuees, wearing tags and carrying their baggage, gathered in groups of around 500 at an appointed place.[4]

The Wartime Civil Control Administration (WCCA) made an effort to take care of any emergency that might arise. A doctor and nurse traveled with each group along with medical supplies and food. The buses stopped as needed, and those who might require medical care were clustered together in one bus with a nurse.[5]

The assembly center lay at the end of their first, but not their final destination. The evacuees left the bus or train, walking to the assembly center between a cordon of armed guards. Seeing the barbed wire and searchlights brought a realization as to their state; they were under guard and considered dangerous. Once inside the gates, some evacuees were searched, fingerprinted, and interrogated. All received inoculations for smallpox and typhoid.[6]

The evacuees were predominantly Buddhist or Protestant. The WCCA's policy allowed evacuees to hold religious services within the center, and they could request assistance from outside religious leaders. The center manager arranged for services and facilities. Caucasian religious workers were not allowed to live in the centers and could visit only by special permit. The church services were monitored for fear they might use propaganda or incitement. Use of the Japanese language was generally prohibited, and written publications had to be cleared.

The ban on speaking Japanese in the centers created a problem for the Buddhists; few priests spoke English. Their services had to be restructured and service materials rewritten.[7]

The physical arrangements of the assembly centers varied according to the previous use of the facility. The racetrack's stalls for horses served as rooms for the evacuees. Exhibition halls on fairgrounds became dining halls, gymnasiums, medical clinics, and warehouses. Army-type barracks were the standard structures hurriedly built to house the evacuees. The barracks were divided into living spaces that could hardly be dignified by the name "rooms." In size they varied from 16 × 20 feet to 20 × 20 feet, depending on the size of the family. Families divided their rooms for modest privacy by hanging sheets if they could be scrounged.[8]

Sounds carried throughout the barracks, as there was no ceiling. It was hard to sleep with babies crying and the sounds of coughing and snoring. Some families argued late in the night. Around fourteen barracks were arranged in blocks, which became the social unit. A block leader, usually an older Issei who had the respect of the group, would be elected. Each block had its own showers, lavatories, and toilets with no partitions. The Japanese, with their passion for cleanliness, found such spartan arrangements and the lack of privacy an embarrassment.[9]

One internee said, "We were always standing in line: eating in the mess hall, using the latrine and waiting for a shower. For us women and children it was such a shock. We got sick…we couldn't go…we didn't want to go. It was smelly and it was dirty. In the showers it was so cramped we almost touched each other. It was humiliating."[10]

The months-long confinement in the unsanitary and crowded makeshift living facilities posed a challenge to the U.S. Public Health Service. Evacuee doctors and nurses were charged with preventing epidemic outbreaks and providing general medical care for the imprisoned population. The recruits found minimal equipment and supplies. One Japanese American evacuee doctor was granted permission to go back to retrieve his instruments, as there were none at the center to help him examine his patients. At Fresno, California, the hospital consisted of one large room with cots. The only supplies were mineral oil, iodine, aspirin, Kaopectate, alcohol, and sulfa ointment.[11]

Although this phase of the incarceration was expected to last only a few weeks, life in the transitory facilities dragged through the long stifling months of summer and into the fall of 1942. The assembly centers were crowded, unhealthy, unsanitary, and demoralizing, and far outlived their intended use. Food handlers were drawn from the common ranks of the evacuees, most of whom had little or no experience working with such vast quantities of food. Their lack of experience conspired with lack of adequate dishwashing and refrigeration equipment, insufficient hot water, incomplete insect screening, and poor sanitation to bring short-term misery to many people.[12]

At the Puyallup Assembly Center a severe outbreak of diarrhea brought on by spoiled Vienna sausages was cause for near panic in the guard towers. Symptoms started at night after everyone was in bed. The limited public latrines were located at some distance, and lighting was poor or nonexistent. People used flashlights to light their way, often to find the latrines already occupied. The guards, seeing a scurry of flashing lights, feared an insurrection was about to take place and called for reinforcements. Order was soon restored, and the epidemic passed without major consequence.[13]

The lack of Nisei nurses necessitated a crash program to train nurse aides. Young women contemplating careers in nursing and any person who wanted to help their fellow man answered the call. Through a series of lectures and demonstrations, student nurse aides learned to make beds, give baths, apply poultices, sterilize equipment and supplies, and provide appropriate infant and maternity care. All centers employed nurse aides because registered nurses were in short supply. Resident medical staffs quickly became dependent upon them.[14]

With a few exceptions, the medical staff treated the usual range of illnesses and injuries. However, there were challenges. At the Santa Anita Assembly Center, hospital records show that about 75 percent of the illnesses came from the occupants of horse stalls. Serious illnesses were treated at nearby hospitals outside the centers, and the Army reported that they paid for these services. Some evacuees, however, recall paying for medical care themselves.[15]

One Japanese American young woman recalls that her family was fortunate in that upon arrival at the San Tanforan Race Track Assembly Center, the horse stalls had all been assigned. The family moved into hastily built barracks. She worked in the mess hall, but she became discouraged because the Caucasian administration and employees skimmed off the best food. She then went to the hospital, enrolled in a nurse aide class, and worked on the medical and communicable disease unit. When it came time to move to a relocation center, she was assigned to the Pullman cars in the transport of mothers with young babies, invalids, stroke patients, the mentally depressed, and the patients recently discharged from hospitals. She was given a lower berth so she could get out easily, but she never had time to sleep there. Instead, she gave her berth to a woman who became ill on the train. Baby formulas were made in the dining room, and the disabled were fed in their bunks. The medical and nursing staff took time to talk to the patients who were apprehensive and fearful of their unknown destination.[16]

The journey took three days, as the train was often sidetracked for a passenger train, a freight train, or a troop train. The medical and nursing staff sat up all night in the sitting rooms because there was no time or place to sleep. Finally, they reached their sandy and windy destination at the Topaz Relocation Center in Utah. Ambulances were waiting to take the patients to the hospital. The woman recalled those days when she reached camp exhausted and slept for two days. She said, "My mother and sister brought food from the mess hall as I was too tired to go myself. After a few days of recuperation I went to the hospital to see how I could help."[17]

Protestant denominations did what they could to ease the trauma of evacuation. Missionaries J.V. and Esther Martin, both Caucasians, had served in Japan before the war years began. In the summer of 1941, they began assisting the Reverend S. Niwa, pastor of the Japanese Methodist Church in Tacoma, Washington. The Martins' primary work was with the English speaking young people, but from the beginning they had cordial relations with the Issei who were born in Japan. The Martins' Christmas letter of 1942 told friends and supporters about their year. From December 7, 1941 to mid-May 1942, church activities went on much as usual, although there were no evening meetings after the curfew. The Federal Bureau of Investigation (FBI) had already taken some of their leading members and imprisoned them in Missoula, Montana. Church attendance increased until the May evacuation. The Martins said that it was the saddest thing they had ever seen and saddest of all was how the Japanese and their American-born children went away smiling. The Tacoma flock was sent to Puyallup Assembly Center where 8,000 were interned, including Japanese Americans from Alaska.[18]

The Martins at first talked to their friends through the barbed wire fence. Later a place was provided just inside the gates where they could visit their Japanese friends at certain hours. The missionaries ran errands for the internees. They brought watches and pens, and took many pairs of shoes for repairs. The Martins also shopped for items such as shoes, shirts, yarn, oranges, slippers, all-day suckers, knitting needles, and soap.[19]

In late August and early September 1942, the Puyallup camp evacuees were moved to their permanent location in Minidoka, Idaho. For several days the Martins went each morning to see them off. They would go up and down each side of the train giving the evacuees flowers that friends had picked from their gardens. Grateful that someone had come to see them off, some wrote letters telling the missionaries how wonderful it was that someone cared enough to come and say goodbye.[20]

When the Puyallup Assembly Center was evacuated, several hospitalized Japanese were left behind, and the Martins visited them weekly. Two died without family and friends to comfort them in their final days. The church used the basement to store household goods for their interned parishioners. As soon as they found out what they could use at the relocation camps, the evacuees wrote for some of their things to be sent to their camp. Some of the requests included curtains that could be used for partitions in their allotted rooms and costumes for a Christmas program.[21]

Evacuees endured the frustrations and hardships for the most part peacefully and stoically. They were told and believed that the assembly centers were temporary. Their hope was for better circumstances on their next move to the relocation centers. In the 1940s young Japanese American women, like their Caucasian peers, were thinking about career options. Many had decided to become nurses while at a young age. Their early desire to devote their lives to a caring profession is evident in their stories. Some had to convince their parents that nursing was an honorable profession. At the outbreak of the war, Sumiko Kumabe Tanouye and Sumiko Ito Dahlman were enrolled in schools of nursing. Kay Shida Tsukuno learned basic nursing skills at a relocation camp and spent seven months caring for her people as a nurse aide. These women at a young age cared for their people during the uprooting, evacuation, and internment of their people during World War II. Their stories follow.

References and Notes

[1] Thomas R. Bodine, *Bodine Papers 1941-1982*. Holdings on Japanese American, Evacuation and Relocation include correspondence, writings, notes, memoranda, reports, newsletters, printed matter, and photographs relating to the relocation of Japanese Americans during World War II, and to the placement of Japanese American students in colleges. Hoover Institution Archives. (Palto Alto, California: Stanford University, No date).

[2] Report of the Commission on Wartime Relocation and Internment of Civilians, *Personal Justice Denied*, (Washington, D.C.: Government Printing Office, 1982):135.

[3] Allen R. Bosworth, *America's Concentration Camps*, (New York: W.W. Norton Company, 1967):113.

[4] Report, 136-7.

[5] Ibid, 136.

[6] Ibid.

[7] Ibid, 145-6.

[8] P. Smith, *Democracy on Trial: Japanese American Evacuation and Relocation In World War II.* (New York: Simon and Schuster, 1995):182-3.

[9] Ibid, 182-3.

[10] Ibid.

[11] Report, 143-4.

[12] Louis Fiset, "Public Health in World War II Assembly Centers for Japanese Americans," *Bulletin of the History of Medicine*, 73 no. 4, Winter, 1999:573.

[13] Ibid.

[14] Ibid, 579.

[15] Ibid.

[16] Anonymous, Nisei Cadet Nurse Project, Boulder, Colorado, 15 May 1999.

[17] Ibid.

[18] Bodine Papers. The J.V. and Esther Martin's Christmas letter. 9 December 1942.

[19] Ibid.

[20] Ibid.

[21] Ibid.

Sumiko Kumabe Tanouye

*Aside from the chaos and uncertainty before me, I was
concerned for the welfare of my family in Hawaii and
with my sisters in Pearl Harbor. There was no means
of communication or any way to gain assurance of their
well-being.*

Sumiko Kumabe Tanouye was born on the Big Island of Hawaii in
1919, as the oldest of seven children to Japanese immigrant parents.
At the turn of the century, in search of a better life, Sumiko's family
immigrated to Hawaii from Kumanmoto, the rural area on the Island
of Kyushu in Japan. As laborers on a sugar plantation in a little community called Hakalau, the Kumabe family toiled on undeveloped land
to grow the best sugar cane that they could, to make enough money to
raise a family, and to own land of their own.

The Japanese culture ingrained the need in Sumiko's parents to
bring up their children in an environment that stressed obedience,
a strong work ethic, and education. Sumiko attended a rural school,
walking miles every morning and returning late in the afternoon on
undeveloped roads. During her seventh and eighth grades she decided
she wanted to be a nurse. In those days, family health care was inad-
equate and often unavailable. The plantation doctor, his apprentices,
and nurses were spread thin and never seemed available in time of need
when illness befell the family. Childhood diseases such as measles,
mumps, and diphtheria were prevalent. Sumiko remembers being quar-
antined in a bedroom and cared for by her family, who carried out the
instructions from the doctor on his daily visits.

Sumiko graduated from Hilo High School in 1938, and her passion to become a nurse grew. At first her parents didn't support Sumiko's ambition. After all, this was a far-fetched dream for the daughter of poor immigrant parents living in rural Hawaii. There were no nursing schools with a college degree program in Hawaii, and 2,000 miles separated her from universities on the West Coast. Sumiko's parents expressed their concern about how their oldest daughter would survive all alone in a far-off land."

Sumiko's parents persuaded her to go to school in Honolulu to become a secretary, which they perceived to be a path toward a safer and more certain future. Reluctantly, she enrolled in a business school in Honolulu, but her heart wasn't in it. After three months she packed her bags and returned home. Sumiko told her parents that typing and office work was not for her. Then she agreed to labor on the plantation to save money in order to attend a university school of nursing in California. Sumiko said, "I worked hard in the fields cutting sugar cane but it wasn't the money that convinced my father to help fund my education and give me permission to leave home. It was my conviction and determination."

Over the years the Kumabe family succeeded in their quest to improve their life compared to the one they had left in Japan. Their family bought land, and Sumiko's father had a good position working for the plantation boss. He was exceptional in that he spoke good English for an immigrant, and his success put him in the position to assist Sumiko in her ambitious endeavors.

Sumiko left Hawaii in the fall of 1939 on the *S.S. Lurline* steamship for a five-day voyage across the Pacific to San Francisco. She continued inland to Sacramento, California and enrolled at the Sacramento Junior College to fulfill prerequisites and earned an associate degree. Two years later she applied at the Children's Hospital in San Francisco and at the University of Chicago's School of Nursing and was accepted at both. She chose the Children's Hospital in San Francisco to be close to relatives in Berkeley and to remain in closer proximity to Hawaii.

Sumiko said, "In the fall of 1941, I began my long-awaited entry into nursing school but, as luck would have it, my nursing training and life took a sudden and unexpected hiatus with the outbreak of war. Aside from the chaos and uncertainty before me, I was concerned for the welfare of my family in Hawaii and with my sisters living in Pearl Harbor. There was no means of communication or any way to gain assurance of their well-being."

Months after the bombing, Sumiko was able to contact her family. Thankfully, everyone was all right. In February of 1942, mass evacuation to internment began. Sumiko's uncle was a semi-invalid and would not survive the conditions of internment. Her relatives were permitted to leave for Denver, Colorado, on a voluntary relocation. Sumiko said, "My family wanted me to join them but I had no means of support. I had gone to the Wells Fargo Bank to withdraw my savings only to learn that my account was frozen and I had only $27 in cash in my purse. My uncle refused to leave without me; I swallowed my pride and accompanied them."

They had 48 hours to pack for the move and were allowed to take only one suitcase for each person. The rest of Sumiko's belongings were packed in boxes and taken to government storage, and she never saw them again. Sumiko said, "I am without pictures and memorabilia of this time."

Sumiko, along with her uncle and cousin's family, traveled to Denver on a slow coal train. Their faces were blackened with soot by the time the miserable journey ended. They were fortunate to have a house pre-arranged in Denver by a cousin. To their disappointment, the inside of the house was bare, with no furniture or bedding. Orange crates served as tables and chairs, and they slept on the floor. As bad as they thought the conditions were at the time, they were thankful that they were all safe and Sumiko's uncle had endured the grueling trip well. In retrospect, they were fortunate to have privacy and their freedom.

Each family member began to look for work, and Sumiko found a job as a live-in housekeeper. The Caucasian family she worked for was kind and understanding, and living with them was pleasant. But she had not lost her determination to complete her nurse training and immediately wrote to the University of Chicago, where she had previously been accepted. Her application was refused because of her ancestry and the outbreak of war.

Rejection only made Sumiko more determined, and she made an appointment at the University of Colorado to learn about the requirements to enroll in the School of Nursing. She enrolled at the University of Colorado's Boulder campus to complete prerequisites at the College of Arts and Sciences. January 1943 she was accepted into the collegiate program of the University of Colorado School of Nursing. She lost credits in the transfer but was all the wiser because of those experiences. Sumiko was happy when her class completed probation and they received their white caps at a capping ceremony.

During Sumiko's second semester, the U.S. Cadet Nurse Corps was instituted and she and her classmates enrolled. This was a great surprise and a happy time for all. Sumiko was especially proud to be recognized in a uniformed service of her country in light of what her people of Japanese ancestry were enduring at this time. She was also proud to inform her father of her newfound self-sufficiency because he had been so supportive of her.

Kay Shida Tsukuno

We were housed in a horse stable at the Santa Anita Racetrack Assembly Center. We filled mattress ticking with straw and slept on the ground. We washed the walls with Lysol to disinfect and to get rid of the odor.

KAY SHIDA TSUKUNO was born and raised in Pasadena, California. Her father came to the United States in 1914. He graduated from high school in Japan but could not speak English when he arrived in this country. He was a farmer and a gardener all of his life. Kay's mother married her father in 1920 at the age of 21. She was a homemaker, worked as a flower grower, and did housework to help provide for the family of three children.

As immigrants the Shida family was segregated within a Japanese community due to the language barrier and support for one another. Kay was bilingual as a young child and served as her parent's interpreter, speaking in Japanese with a sprinkling of English words. Kay's parents emphasized getting an education and encouraged their children to reach their goals. Kay concentrated on her English speaking skills and regrets not becoming proficient in the Japanese language.

Executive Order 1099 disrupted the Shida family's peaceful life. They were given three days to get their affairs in order and to put essential items in one suitcase. They sold their furniture, automobile, and they gave away treasured possessions to neighbors. "We were afraid of what the future held for us," Kay reflected. "We did not know where we were going or what would happen to us. It was hard to understand why Japan attacked the United States and that we had to suffer for their aggression."

Kay remembers, "We were housed in a horse stable at the Santa Anita Racetrack Assembly Center. We filled mattress ticking with straw and slept on the ground. We were issued a pie tin with a fork and spoon, as knives were considered contraband. We washed the walls with Lysol to disinfect and to get rid of the odor."

Wanting to be of service to her people, Kay volunteered to train as a nurse aide. Kay's interest in nursing was sparked early in her life when her brother was hospitalized for possible surgery for a brain tumor. The tumor was inoperable, and he developed seizures and died in his early 20s. His illness gave Kay the desire and incentive to become a nurse in order to care for others. Kay worked as an aide in the Santa Anita makeshift infirmary and saw her first delivery.

Kay and her family, under military guard, were taken by train from California to the Jerome Relocation Center in Arkansas, 25 miles north of the Louisiana border. The family of five shared a room in their assigned barrack. Meals were eaten in the community mess hall, and bathroom facilities were shared by block neighbors. For seven months Kay worked as a nurse aide in the camp hospital staffed by two Japanese American doctors and lab technicians. In the spring of 1943 Kay received FBI clearance and was released under the sponsorship of the Franciscan diocese. She continued to work as an aide at St. Mary's hospital in St. Louis, Missouri and began her search for a school of nursing that would accept her. Kay applied to many Midwestern and Eastern schools but none would consider her application.

In 1943 the University of Minnesota lifted the ban on Japanese American students. The School of Nursing admitted six Japanese American students who were subjected to certain stipulations: (1) Could the Nisei students work with instructors?, (2) Could the Japanese Americans get along with other students?, and (3) Would the patients accept the Nisei students? Kay was approached by a U.S. Cadet Nurse Corps representative and she signed up for the duration of the war.

After successfully completing the student nurse probationary period, Kay remembers the day she was "capped" and the camaraderie of her class that continues 50 years later. She vividly recalls an incident while she was on the graveyard shift as a junior cadet. She discovered a small elderly patient missing from his bed and searched frantically. Then Kay discovered he had crawled into bed with another patient. What a relief!

Kay was taught by Sister Kenny the method of applying hot packs which relieved the terrible pain caused by polio and how to assist recovering patients in their range-of-motion exercises. Sister Kenny was known as the "polio messiah from Australia." Kay was awed by her dedication, knowledge, and love for those stricken with polio-myelitis. Kay also admired and respected Katherine Densford, the elegant and distinguished Dean of Nursing who was also President of the American Nurses Association at this time. Densford was the first woman to be appointed Dean at the University of Minnesota.

As a senior cadet, Kay's visiting nurse rotation took her to Davenport, Iowa—a heart-wrenching experience. Here she cared for patients living in poverty, an experience she will never forget. With her

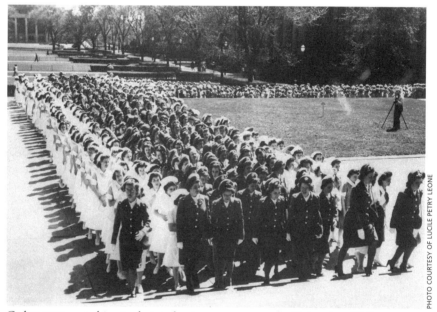

Cadet nurses marching to their induction ceremony at the University of Minnesota School of Nursing, May 13, 1944.

parents interned and no other source of help, it would have been difficult to obtain an education without the U.S. Cadet Nurse Corps.

After the war, Kay exchanged her cadet nurse uniform for the all-white which she proudly wore to her graduation from the University of Minnesota School of Nursing in June of 1950. Kay said, "My mother often told us that this is our adopted country and we must obey the laws. After World War II, my parents studied and took the examination to become naturalized citizens. This was a happy day in their lives."

Kay is proud to be an alumni of the Minnesota University School of Nursing. Here is an excerpt from her alumni newsletter written by an anonymous cadet nurse.

> There were so many new choices a woman could make in 1943. But one choice was obvious. The University of Minnesota. It had always been there, a symbol of strength and excellence. I was proud of my country. Proud of the uniform I wore. And proud that the training I got at the University let me make a difference. The University prepared me for life. And helped me make the right choices, then and throughout my life. I am still proud of my Minnesota University School of Nursing.

Sumiko Ito Dahlman

The bedridden patients were apprehensive as to where we were going and what would happen when we got there. I walked up and down the aisles of the train trying to allay the patients' fears, not knowing what lay ahead for myself.

Sumiko Ito Dahlman grew up in the International District of Seattle, Washington. Her father was a photographer, and her mother was a seamstress. Sumiko had a brother and a sister, and their parents often took them to the beaches, parks, and zoo. The family enjoyed visiting with their Japanese friends who had arrived from the same prefectures in Japan as their parents.

Since early school days, Sumiko wanted to be a nurse, but her parents thought the work would be too strenuous. Seeing her determination, they relented and Sumiko entered the University of Washington to major in nursing. In the spring of 1942 her course of study was interrupted when she and her family were interned first at the Puyullap Assembly Center. They found rows and rows of hastily built tarpaper barracks surrounded by barbed wire, wooden watch towers, searchlights, and armed military police. The family of five shared one room, that was 10×18 feet with no furniture. They were given bags to fill with straw for mattresses.

Sumiko volunteered to work as a nurse aide for six months when the evacuees were notified that they would be moved to a relocation center (they did not know where). Sumiko volunteered to stay behind with the hospital team to assist in the transport of the bedridden patients. The patients were brought to the train on stretchers and lifted through the windows of the train, then placed on bunks. The team worked in four-hour shifts, and Sumiko had some narrow escapes managing trays and bedpans on the lurching train. One of Sumiko's patients had delivered a baby just a few days before they left. She had a difficult time conveying to the dining room staff that she needed to sterilize bottles and mix formula.

"The bedridden patients were apprehensive as to where they were going and what would happen when we got there," Sumiko said. "I walked up and down the aisles of the train trying to allay the patients' fears, not knowing what lay ahead for myself." One patient was a paraplegic and could not talk. Sumiko stayed close and talked to her.

The Minidoka Relocation Center in Idaho was the Ito family's destination. Sumiko recalls that the facilities were somewhat improved, but the family continued to shared one room. Summers were hot with dust storms, and winters were cold with deep snow. Sumiko's father's background in photography qualified him to work in the X-Ray department at the hospital. Her brother, a math major, taught math in the camp school, and her younger sister was enrolled in grade school.

Sumiko continued to work as a nurse aide but found her situation stagnating; she desperately wanted to leave camp. The protocol for leaving was acceptance at a school or to have a job in an inland state. She filled out countless applications with discouraging replies such as, "Dear Miss Ito: We are sorry but our quota is full."

The happy day finally arrived when Sumiko received her acceptance letter from the St. Mary's Hospital School of Nursing in Rochester, Minnesota. After reviewing her papers, the War Relocation Authority sanctioned her leaving camp. One day a representative came to St. Mary's and told Sumiko and her peers about the U.S. Cadet Nurse Corps. Without hesitation, Sumiko joined the Corps. During her second year, Sumiko found a job for her father, and her parents were able to join her in Minneapolis.

As a senior cadet nurse, Sumiko was assigned to serve in the Schick General Army Hospital in Clinton, Iowa. Here they wore the cadet nurse uniform while off duty and the hospital uniform of her school, with the Maltese patch, when working on the wards. Sumiko said,

"Being a part of the Cadet Nurse Corps helped us to become better citizens. We were proud of our insignia, and we did our best to uphold the Corps."

5 Cities Behind Barbed Wire

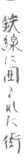

On April 7, 1942, Milton S. Eisenhower, director of the War Relocation Authority, met with ten governors or their representatives from ten western states—Arizona, Colorado, Idaho, Montana, New Mexico, Nevada, Oregon, Utah, Washington, and Wyoming—to discuss a plan for resettlement for the people of Japanese ancestry. His idea was to set up 50 to 75 small inland camps similar to the Civilian Conservation Corps camps, a successful program during the days of the Great Depression. From the small camps the evacuees would be moved out as rapidly as possible to places other than the West Coast. Eisenhower explained that none of the evacuees had been charged with disloyalty, and they had been evacuated as a defense measure.[1]

In his later memoirs, Eisenhower said that he planned to discuss policies regarding wages, health care, and other factors but got no further. The governors and representatives had been deaf to Eisenhower's opening assurance. They began shouting and shaking their fists in his face arguing that if these people were considered dangerous on the Pacific Coast, they would be dangerous in the Midwest as well.[2]

Only Governor Ralph Carr of Colorado took a reasonable position. He said he had no objections to having loyal Japanese Americans moving into his state and that cooperation with the relocation project was a citizen's responsibility. He was the single exception. Eisenhower had hoped that the governors would make it possible for the people to resettle in their states, to be given the chance to live normally and to contribute to the communities.[3]

Disappointed, Eisenhower said that there was no alternative but to create confinement centers where people could live in modest comfort, do useful work, have schools for the children, and maintain as much self-respect as the horrible circumstances permitted. The search for the relocation centers proceeded during April and into May 1942. The sites had to be large enough to accommodate a small city of 8,000 or more. The sites also needed to be located away from strategic installations but with a potential of providing useful work opportunities.[4]

Near the end of May 1942, the first evacuees began to arrive at the relocation centers. They had been assured that the War Relocation

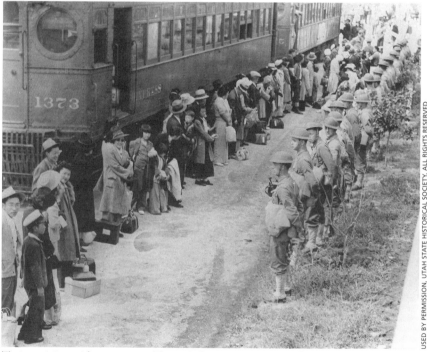

Train arriving with evacuees at Topaz Relocation Center, Utah, population 10,000.

Authority camps would better meet their families' needs than the assembly centers. The evacuees also believed that some of the repressive elements of the assembly centers, particularly the guard towers and barbed wire, would be eliminated. They were prepared for an orderly, cooperative move.[5]

The ten sites selected, however, were unattractive and inhospitable. Manzanar and Poston, already selected by the Army, were in the deserts of California and Arizona. Six other sites were also in arid desert. Gila River, near Phoenix, suffered from intense heat. The two most northern centers, Minidoka in Idaho and Heart Mountain in Wyoming, were known for harsh winters and dust storms. Tule Lake, in north-central California, was located in a dry lake bed. Utah's Topaz was covered with greasewood, and Colorado's Amache was in the middle of a dry, parched, windswept prairie dotted by sagebrush and yucca. The Arkansas sites were entirely different. These camps were heavily wooded, snake-infested swamplands. The new confinement centers where evacuees would be arriving were hardly improved over the assembly centers.[6]

The policy at the relocation centers stated that the evacuees would receive food, shelter, medical care, and education without charge. In the relocation centers evacuees were given the opportunity to work. Doctors, dentists, nurses, and teachers were at the top of the pay scale, earning $19 a month. The majority of workers received $16, and apprentices and nurse aides earned $12. Meager as it was, the evacuees needed the money and chose to work.[7]

Many could not afford to order even the barest of essentials from the Sears Roebuck catalogue. Shoes for growing children were out of reach. Some evacuees saw no reason to give their efforts toward a system that had displayed so little trust in them. Despite these problems, the centers were staffed almost completely by the evacuees. Workers were needed in food preparation, winterization, health and sanitation, security, and schools. The evacuees set about making the best of a despairing situation.[8]

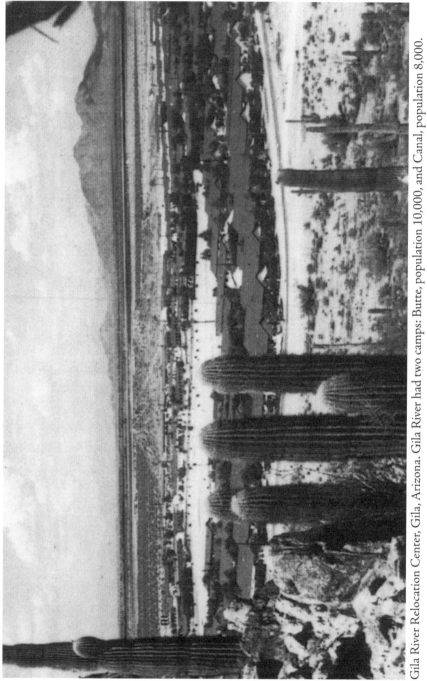

Gila River Relocation Center, Gila, Arizona. Gila River had two camps: Butte, population 10,000, and Canal, population 8,000.

The eviction and detention of Japanese American orphans is another story. Prior to the U.S. involvement in the war and the evacuation orders that followed, Japanese American orphans resided in three California orphanages. Within days of Japan's attack on Pearl Harbor the Federal Bureau of Investigation began detaining "suspect" Japanese and Japanese Americans. The Bureau's arrest directly impacted the lives of Japanese American children and orphans.[9]

Janice Matsuko Kaku was born in San Francisco, California, where her parents ran a grocery store. She was 13 years of age when her parents died, and Janice and her sisters were placed in a Japanese orphanage in Silver Lake, California. There the Matsuko sisters attended public schools. Shortly after December 7, 1941, Janice and her sisters were sent home from school because of the curfew. Janice said that this time was the saddest in her young life.[10]

The incarceration of alien Japanese orphanage workers left no one to care for the children during the war. The government proposed dispersing the orphans throughout the different camps. Harry and Lillian Matsumoto, directors of one of the orphanages in the Los Angeles area, strongly favored keeping the children together in an effort to maintain some familiarity and structure. The idea of an orphanage within a camp was conceived and in April 1942, the Matsumotos and personnel from the California Child Welfare Department visited the Manzanar Relocation site to see if this arrangement would be feasible. The Children's Village opened its doors on June 23, 1942. The Matsumotos were named directors and given the authority to operate the orphanage as they saw fit.[11]

Since the barracks provided for the evacuees were unsuitable for young children, three one-story buildings were built by the evacuees. They were of better quality, (wider and stronger) and complete with running water, toilets, and laundry facilities.[12] Janice and her three sisters were among 101 American orphans of Japanese ancestry interned for either a period of time or the duration of the war during the Children's Village existence. The Children's Village was a camp within a camp.

Two Japanese American recent high school graduates, Chiyeko Inashima and Katsuko Kato Odanaka describe their feelings upon their arrival to their particular city (Minidoka and Manzanar) behind barbed wire. Both Chiyeko and Katsuko turned a dismal situation into a beginning step toward their future profession in nursing. They enrolled in a nurse aide training course and used their skills in helping to staff relocation hospitals in Idaho and California. This training and experience would help open further doors for Chiyeko and Katsuko in gaining entrance to a school of nursing.

References and Notes

[1] Bill Hosokawa, *Nisei, The Quiet Americans: The Story of a People*, (New York: Doubleday & Company, Inc., 1969):338.

[2] Milton S. Eisenhower. *The President is Calling*, (Garden City, New York: Doubleday & Company, Inc., 1974):118.

[3] Ibid, 120.

[4] Ibid.

[5] Report of the Commission on Wartime Relocation and Internment of Civilians, *Personal Justice Denied*, (Washington, D. C):GPO, 1982):3.

[6] Ibid, 156-8.

[7] Valerie Matsumoto, "Japanese American Women During World War II," *Frontiers* 8, no. 1 (1984):9.

[8] Report, 167-8.

[9] Lisa N. Nove, "The Children's Village at Manzanar: The World War II Eviction and Detention of Japanese American Orphans," *Journal of the West* 38, no. 2 (April 1999), 65-68.

[10] Janice Matsuko Kodani Karu, Nisei Cadet Nurse Project, Boulder, Colorado, 28 February 2001.

[11] Nove.

[12] J. Burton, M. Farrell, F. Lord, and R. Lord, "Manzanar Relocation Center, Chapter 8," *Confinement and Ethnicity: An Overview of World War II Japanese American Relocation Sites*, National Park Service, 2000, Park Net www.cr.nps.gov/hist/online.

Chiyeko Inashima

*Small children started to cry and said they wanted to go
home. We felt sorry for the mothers, but I think all of us
could have cried.*

CHIYEKO INASHIMA was born and raised in Seattle, Washington, and
her family lived in a community that was mainly Oriental. An area of
about 24 blocks comprised the Japanese community. China Town was
a block away with a scattering of Filipinos living among them. A few
Black families also lived in the community. Chiyeko's parents' lives were
occupied by working for a living and raising their children to become
upright citizens. They wanted their children to remember their heritage
and sent them to Japanese language school.

Growing up, Chiyeko loved reading stories about nurses. The deeds
of bravery and good works of Clara Barton, Florence Nightingale,
and Lillian Wald fascinated her. On her way to school she passed two
hospitals and admired the nurses going to work in their white uniforms
and blue capes. One day Chiyeko announced to her parents that she
was going to be a nurse. They were appalled and told her that no girl in
their family was going to be a nurse nor would she go to college. They
added that nurses were degraded persons and that college spoiled girls.
Chiyeko kept her ambition to herself and would years later prove them
wrong.

Soon after the Executive Order 9066 was signed in February of
1942 an announcement came that volunteer movement away from
the Pacific Coast was permitted. The Inashima family, like most other
families, knew no one inland and chose to stay and let the government
take action The city was divided into areas, and they were not allowed

to step foot outside their prescribed region. When the 8 p.m. curfew was imposed, anyone outside of their homes was arrested. Chiyeko, a senior in high school, would graduate in June. Getting to school and attending school functions became difficult and at times impossible.

The Inashima family's section of the city was scheduled for evacuation in early May. The Seattle schools assured the Japanese American students that they would receive credit for the semester. Chiyeko regretted missing out on the senior prom and all of the graduation activities. The principal of her high school and the president of the student body obtained special permission to come to the Puyallup Assembly Center. They conducted a special high school graduation exercise, in which Chiyeko and her senior class friends received their diplomas.

Each area at the assembly center was enclosed with a high barbed wire fence with posted guard towers. The front gate was manned by two armed guards, and only those with passes were allowed in or out. The assembly centers were temporarily built of the cheapest of materials. The knots in the wood fell out, and families could peer into the quarters next door as well as get a peek of the outside.

On Sundays a minister from Seattle came to conduct services. Each Sunday a different denomination would hold services in a different area of the center. The internees lined up in front of the gate, and armed guards escorted them to the area where church services were held. Leaving their restricted area gave them the opportunity to see friends confined in another area.

In September of 1942 Chiyeko and her family were told that they were moving out to permanent quarters and to pack their belongings. The group was bused to the depot, where they boarded a dilapidated train for their unknown destination. Shades were drawn, and they were ordered to not touch the shades. After a stifling ride of a couple of days, the train stopped and they were informed that they were at their final destination.

Chiyeko recalled:

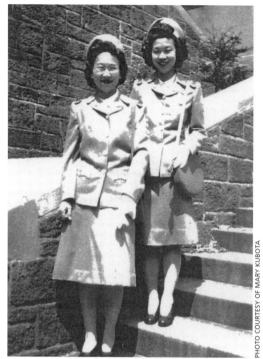

Mary Kubota (left) and Chiyeko Inashima in
cadet nurse uniform. Bellevue School of Nursing,
New York City.

I shall never forget the moment we stepped off the train and sank into dry sand that came up to our ankles. We looked around and saw nothing but tumbling tumble weeds. The wind blew sand into our eyes and we were unable to see. Small children started to cry and said they wanted to go home. We felt sorry for the mothers, but I think all of us could have cried.

Military guards checked evacuees as they boarded a bus that took them to another barbed wire enclosed area. The guards escorted the internees into the enclosed area, then the Inashima family was led to a barrack and given their assigned quarters. At this time they were informed that they were at the Minidoka Relocation Center in Idaho.

To while away their boredom, most evacuees volunteered to work. Chiyeko's mother worked as a cleaning woman at the hospital, and

Chiyeko took the nurse aide training and worked on the hospital wards. One day an announcement was made that college students could return to their studies providing they could find a sponsor. Chiyeko began filling out form after form. Chiyeko's church and two former Sunday school teachers agreed to sponsor her. Chiyeko said that to this day she is grateful and thankful for their kind gesture.

In February 1943, Chiyeko and four other Nisei students were on their way to freedom and traveled together as far as Omaha, Nebraska. Entirely on her own in an unknown world, Chiyeko arrived in Kansas City, Missouri, but was devastated by the news that her course would not be offered until fall. Chiyeko did not want to return to camp and wired her brother, now attending the University of Idaho in Pocatello, for assistance. He contacted the Dean, who sent a letter asking Chiyeko to send transcripts and credentials from the schools she had attended and to be there in two weeks.

Chiyeko returned to Idaho, but this time for a more awarding experience to attend the University. At the end of her freshmen year she learned about the U.S. Cadet Nurse Corps, switched her major to pre-nursing and began searching for a school of nursing. The prestigious Bellevue School of Nursing in New York City accepted her application. Chiyeko remembers attending four hours of classes each day then working on the wards during the evening or night shift. With the war going on, supplies were hard to obtain and as a cadet nurse she learned to improvise. "We learned self-reliance and responsibility in a hurry and were taught where to go for answers when we needed them," Chiyeko said.

In spite of her parents not wanting her to be a nurse or to get an education, Chiyeko received a bachelor of science in nursing and a master's degree in occupational health and safety. She also fulfilled her commitment to the government that interned her and her family by serving as a nurse for the duration of World War II. The U.S. Cadet Nurse Corps in turn provided her the beginning of a lifetime education—free.

Katsuko Kato Odanaka

The internees who had arrived before us were lined up looking us over, trying to find a familiar face.

KATSUKO KATO ODANAKA's parents, first generation immigrants from Okayama-ken, Japan, supported themselves by going into various businesses in Los Angeles. They had no other relatives in this country. The community in which Katsuko grew up had many Japanese families. As Buddhists, the Kato family attended services and participated in various festivals. Oban Festival was celebrated with a street parade. The women dressed in kimonos and wore crowns on their heads.

New Year's Day was a special celebration for the Japanese community. Katsuko's father invited friends for a *moche-tsuki* (the pounding of rice in a large concrete bowl with big wooden mallets). Rice was pounded until mushy, and then formed into patties for a special New Year's dish. Her mother prepared an elaborate assortment of Japanese food and dishes. Each year the family attended a Kenji Wi Kai picnic, enjoying friends from the same area in which her parents grew up. Nisei Week Festival in Lil' Tokyo was an annual event for the Japanese community. A queen and her attendants were selected, followed with street dancing in kimonos and happy jackets.

The schools Katsuko attended were racially mixed with Latinos, Blacks, Asians, and Caucasians, and there was little racial conflict. Katsuko attended Japanese school every day after her regular school day. After Katsuko's parents converted to Christianity, they attended worship service and Sunday school. Their church provided a strong support group for her family.

After the Pearl Harbor attack, there was continuous news about the possibility of evacuation of all those with Japanese ancestry, regardless of citizenship, living on the West Coast. Katsuko was in the 11th grade, attending Jefferson High School, when Executive Order 9066 was announced. Public notices were posted in all Japanese communities. Announcements were also made on the radio, in churches, and by Japanese community leaders. Photographic equipment was confiscated before evacuation. They were directed to meet at a certain location, then bused to the trains. With minimum luggage and belongings they boarded the train for an unknown life and destination.

Several days later the Kato family found themselves at the gate of the Manzanar Relocation Center. It was located in a desolate, dusty area in eastern California. "The camp was surrounded by barbed wire fence with guard towers to confine us," Katsuko remembered. "The evacuees who had arrived before us were lined up looking us over, trying to find a familiar face."

The new residents were issued canvas bags to fill with straw for their mattresses and given blankets. Their assigned room had a wood-burning stove, and blankets were hung for privacy when they could spare them. All evacuees ate in the mess hall staffed by camp residents, and they used communal restrooms. Eventually, schools were established, and there were churches of all faiths, community activities, movies, dancing, and sports events. Manzanar had a population of 10,000.

After some time, camp life became organized and settled. Life was fairly pleasant for Katsuko's age group. With lots of young people to associate with, they enjoyed participating in after-school activities. Katsuko said that her teachers were great and related to their needs. After graduating from Manzanar High School, Katsuko took the nurse aide training and worked at the camp hospital.

A difficult time occurred when the residents were required to sign a loyalty oath to the U.S. government. Many Nisei, American citizens by birth, resented their government making such a demand after the treatment they had received. Their parents, the Issei, were not permitted to become U.S. citizens. The Kibeis were second generation Japanese

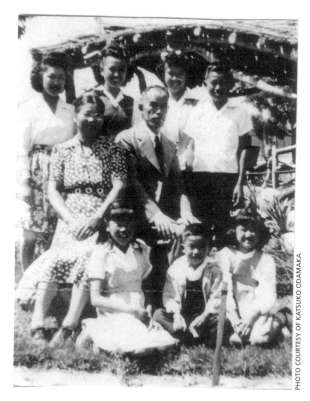

Kato Family at
Manzanar Camp, 1945.

"Pleasure Park" in
Manzanar. The Kato
family poses on a
bridge in a Japanese
garden built by
evacuees, 1943.

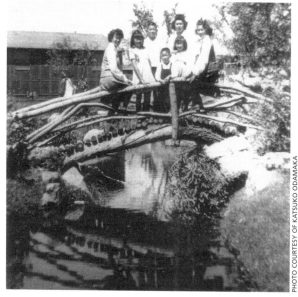

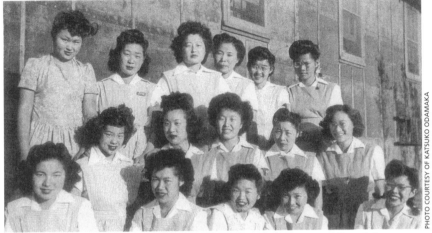

Nurse Aides at Manzanar Camp Hospital, 1944. Katsuko is second from left.

who had returned to Japan for education and extended visits with relatives. These young people had pleasant memories and affections for their motherland. Families were divided between those signing the oath and those who refused. The resisters who failed to sign the oath were moved out of Manzanar to a more secured camp in Northern California. Fortunately for Katsuko, her family members all signed the oath.

After Katsuko obtained her security clearance, she was permitted to travel to Chicago, Illinois, to pursue a nursing career. The War Relocation Authority (WRA) had offices in various cities to assist evacuees in their resettlement. They advised Katsuko as to the schools of nursing accepting Japanese American students. The WRA arranged for her to work as a nurse aide at a retirement home in Evanston, Illinois. The cook and several other nurse aides were also Japanese Americans. Katsuko missed her family and friends back in camp, but the transition went well.

In July of 1945 Katsuko was accepted by the Evangelical Deaconess Hospital School of Nursing, located in an Irish-Polish neighborhood in Chicago. She did not encounter prejudice during her three years of training. Her classmates invited Katsuko and another Nisei nurse student into their homes and included them in activities outside of the nursing school.

After graduation Katsuko continued to work in the hospital where she trained as an obstetrics and delivery room charge nurse. Four years later, Katsuko returned to Los Angeles, California. She worked as an operating room nurse and met her husband, Woodrow Odanako in 1951. Katsuko took a break from nursing while she cared for her four young children. The family moved to Whittier, California and she returned to nursing in 1966. After 22 years, Katsuko retired from her position as nurse administrator. She said, "I will always be grateful for the Cadet Nurse Corps for paying my nursing school expenses as my parents were still in camp and unable to help me financially."

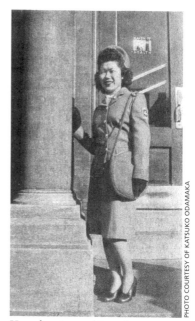

Katsuko pictured in cadet nurse uniform.

⑥ Life in Camp

収
容
所
生
活

Several nights ago a guard shot a cow...the guard responsible verified it. While he was walking back and forth at night all by himself, he noticed something moving by the fence. He shouted "Halt!" and repeated, "Halt!" Then he fired twice. The poor cow had to be butchered. The guards had orders to shoot to kill. What would have happened if some thoughtless child tried to climb through the fence to retrieve a ball or pick a flower?

        – Letter written by an interned university student.[1]

T HE EVACUEES INTERNED AT the assembly centers were under the Army jurisdiction. When they were moved to the relocation centers, they came under the custody of a new agency: the War Relocation Authority (WRA). Military police continued to patrol the perimeters of the camps monitoring entries and exits. The high fences and the presence of the guards signified their continued loss of freedom and independence.

Author Yoshiko Uchida writes about her experience:

> We often took walks along the edge of camp, watching sunsets made spectacular by the dusty haze and waiting for the moon to rise in the

darkening sky. It was one of the few things to look forward to in our life at Topaz.

Sometimes as we walked, we could hear the Military Police singing in their quarters, and then they seemed something more than sentries who patrolled the barbed wire perimeters of our camp, and we realized they were lonely young boys far from home too. Still, they were on the other side of the fence, and they represented the Army we had come to fear and distrust. We never offered them our friendship, although at times they tried to talk to us.[2]

The working wages of $12, $16, or $19 per month, plus a clothing allowance for dependent members of family averaging $3 per month, was hardly adequate. The families could only take what they could carry, and the evacuees sent to cold climates were not prepared for the harsh weather. In spite of primitive laundry facilities, the internees always appeared neat and clean. Limited wardrobes received hard wear, which was especially true for shoes. The centers had no sidewalks, and the streets were rough with gravel and stones.[3]

When the evacuees began arriving at the relocation centers, the education program was little more than a promise. School buildings were not part of the Army base style of construction so classes were held in barracks. In the beginning, sometimes the teacher had a desk and a chair, but more often it was just a chair and the children sat on the floor. Equipment was always hard to come by. The students in a typing class at Tule Lake never saw a typewriter. They drew circles on sheets of papers, lettered the circles, and practiced pressing their fingers on the circles. At Minidoka washrooms became biology and chemistry laboratories.

States began donating old textbooks and other donations came from the American Friends Service Committee in Philadelphia, Pennsylvania. Education at four different levels included nursery school, elementary school, high school, and adult education. The curriculum was consistent with the state education requirements in which the camp was located. All schools except Tule Lake were accredited. Ironically, education programs emphasized "Americanization." A before-school ritual included giving the pledge of allegiance and singing, "My country, 'tis of thee, sweet land of liberty." Caucasian teachers found the ceremony awkward and embarrassing in the austere prison-camp settings.[4]

The camps were busy places. Most of the evacuees who could work did so, and they worked with the WRA to create the illusion of a normal community. Nowhere was this more evident than in the evacuees' efforts to set up community activities. Throughout internment there are stories of ingenuity, resourcefulness, endurance, and patience as to how the evacuees' dealt with mass segregation.[5] Camp life increased the leisure time for the Issei who had worked so hard all of their lives. The women, especially, found that the communally prepared meals and limited living quarters gave them spare time. Many availed themselves of the opportunities to attend adult classes taught by both evacuees and non-Japanese. Courses included handcrafts in the traditional Japanese arts such as flower arrangement, sewing, painting, calligraphy, and wood carving. Many turned to art for self-expression.[6]

In the relocation centers there were no government funds for social, religious, and recreational activities. Church groups came through with donated equipment. While preferences of Issei and Nisei differed, baseball was a common denominator for teams ranging in ages from 6 to 60. Most of the centers had libraries. Holidays were celebrated. Arbor Day was observed in Topaz with the distribution of small shrubs for each block. At Christmas there were special foods, decorations and presents donated by the American Friends Society. New Year's was celebrated traditionally with *mochi*, a kind of rice cake. Easter was celebrated with large outdoor ceremonies. Buddhists held parades and folk dances to celebrate the anniversary of the birth of Buddha. The WRA did not pay ministers and priests, so they were financed by congregations and national churches. Unlike in the assembly centers, here the speaking of Japanese was permitted.[7]

In Colorado, the residents of the Granada Relocation Center referred to their camp as Amache, named after the daughter of Cheyenne Chief Ochi-Nee who lived in the area. The patriotic spirit of this group prevailed throughout internment. The boy scouts organized a paper drive. Scrap metal was also collected. A president's ball was held with proceeds going to the March of Dimes. An Amache victory concert raised money for victory bonds and stamps. In late 1943 the Red Cross set a goal to raise $500 and netted $1,200. The boys and girls in the Future Farmers of America grew victory gardens. The Amache Blue Star Mothers Club sponsored dances to entertain soldiers on furlough. A silk screen shop manufactured Navy training posters and produced 60,000 between 1943 and 1944.[8]

In January 1943, antagonists declared that evacuees were being coddled, and the WRA ordered the centers to submit menus for each 30-day period. Food for the evacuees could cost no more than rations for the Army, which was set at 50¢ per person per day. The actual costs per evacuee fell below that cost, and no appetizing meals could be produced regularly under such a requirement. The best that could be said for the meal system at the camps is that no one starved.[9]

No one froze either. When winter first approached many evacuees were unprepared for cold weather due to baggage limitations. Having formerly lived in warmer climates they did not possess adequate clothing. Army surplus distribution became the principal source of warm clothing during that first winter. Old sailor pea jackets and GI uniforms, sizes 38 to 44, were handed out. At least they were warm and the oversized garments became the source of great amusement.[10]

In signing Executive Order 9066, President Franklin Roosevelt had succumbed to political and military pressure. Eleanor Roosevelt was shaken when the news reached her, according to Doris Kearns Goodwin. She had witnessed the growing hysteria toward the Japanese living in our country and feared that something like this might happen. She tried to speak to her husband, but he gave her a frigid reception and said not to mention the subject again.[11]

In April 1943 President Roosevelt received a letter from Interior Secretary Harold Ickes suggesting that there was unrest in the Japanese internment camps, creating hostile groups on the home front. Eleanor Roosevelt served unofficially as the president's eyes and ears, and now he asked the First Lady to check out the situation. Arriving at Gila River Relocation Center on April 23, 1943, Mrs. Roosevelt encountered the swirling dust that left everyone's hair white, mouths gritty, and eyes red.[12]

Dillon Myer, the present director of the War Relocation Authority, escorted Mrs. Roosevelt through the camp. Myer was amazed at her tireless energy. She wanted to see everything of any importance, including all of the wards of the hospital, the schools, and all phases of the service activities so she could report back to the President. She left with a deep respect for the ingenuity and endurance of the Japanese. Despite the wind and the dust, she found a productive community. Among the internees were many experienced produce growers, and they had tapped into the canal water, turning the desert wasteland into a lush, productive farmland and supplying the kitchens with fresh vegetables and melons of all sorts. Pigs thrived on garbage from the camp and then the residents ate the pigs. Chickens provided eggs and meat, and cattle supplied milk and beef. A camouflage net factory was producing far beyond expectations.[13]

"Everything is spotlessly clean," Mrs. Roosevelt reported. She marveled at small Japanese gardens with vegetables and flowers and the makeshift porches and shades improvised with gunny sacks and bits of wood salvaged from packing crates. But she recognized that there was a breakdown of the traditional family structure. With the thousands of people assembled together, parents were unable to exercise control or influence over their children. Mrs. Roosevelt determined that the only answer was to relax the exclusion order and to allow the Japanese to return to their homes "to start independent and productive lives again." Dillon Myer agreed.[14]

Alice Noguchi Kanagaki will never forget the day Mrs. Roosevelt visited Gila River Relocation Camp in Arizona. Her story follows.

References and Notes

[1] Thomas R. Bodine, *Bodine Papers 1941-1982*, Hoover Institution Archives, (Palo Alto, California: Stanford University.) Selection from evacuation stories, no date.

[2] Yoshiko Uchida, *Desert Exile: The Uprooting of a Japanese American Family*, (Seattle: University of Washington Press, 1982):112.

[3] Report of the Commission on Wartime Relocation and Internment of Civilians, *Personal Justice Denied*, (Washington, D.C.: Government Printing Office, 1982):170-3.

[4] Ibid.

[5] Ibid.

[6] Valerie Matsumoto, "Japanese American Women During World War II," *Frontiers* 8, no. 1 (1948):9.

[7] Report, 172-3.

[8] Dean A. Swartz, "Patriotism Amidst Prejudice: The Irony, Individuality and Impact of Patriotism at Amache," (honors thesis, University of Colorado, 1979):5-6.

[9] Ibid.

[10] Report, 163.

[11] Ibid, 323-3.

[12] Doris Kerns Goodwin, *No Ordinary Time Franklin and Eleanor Roosevelt: The Home Front in World War II*, (New York: Simon and Schuster, 1994):427.

[13] Ibid.

[14] Ibid.

Alice Noguchi Kanagaki

*We were situated on the reservation grounds of the Gila
River Indian community, home of the Pima and Maricopa
tribes, and there were frequent visits from the Native
Americans. The Indians came riding in buckboards and on
horseback to view us with much curiosity. Later friendships
were formed, and some sports competition ensued.*

ALICE NOGUCHI KANAGAKI and her three older brothers grew up in
the rural community of Vacaville, California. Fruit farming was the
mainstay of the town's industries, and one could refer to some of the
owners as land barons. They lived in large Victorian mansions and
possessed hundreds, and sometimes nearly thousands, of acres of fruit
orchards. Alice's father rented a portion of an orchard, and at the end
of the harvest season, he paid the rental fee and the workers; anything
remaining was the family's meager share.

Vacaville was a community of about 1,500 people with an interesting mixture of Caucasians, Hispanics, Japanese, and a few Chinese. The
Hispanics had their own church and social activities. The Japanese had
both Methodist and Buddhist religions. The Japanese language and
martial arts were taught in the large Buddhist building. The Noguchis
attended the Methodist church, a smaller congregation whose minister
served several rural communities. The Japanese church provided most
of the social activities, such as holiday parties and picnics.

All of the town's people attended school activities such as intercity
sports, school plays, and graduation ceremonies. Alice's brothers were
Boy Scouts, and Alice participated in the Drum and Bugle Corps. Her
group performed in parades and events in neighboring towns and were

invited to march in the opening day parade of the World's Fair, held in 1939 on Treasure Island in San Francisco, California.

Though everyone was recovering from the depression years, growing up in the 1930s was a bountiful time for the Noguchi family of six. Crime against children was rare. Children walked and biked out in the country, and people did not hesitate to pick up hitchhikers. Alice and her cousin, along with their dogs, explored creeks, wooded hills, and open fields, picking and smelling the many wildflowers that could be found in the California outdoors. In springtime, the acres and acres of flowering fruit trees gave the entire countryside a wonderful fragrance. Each year the Noguchi family packed a scrumptious picnic lunch and drove into the orchards, where they spread blankets and savored the warm sunshine, the aroma from the flowering fruit trees, and song birds.

While the Noguchi family was poor, they never lacked for food, as they had vegetable gardens, chickens, and eggs. Alice said that the chickens were like pets that most of the family ate without qualms; her mother, however, was attached to the pets, alive or cooked. Alice's mother was a wonderful cook, made nearly all of Alice's clothes, and gave her children haircuts. She taught them good manners, pride, and to do their best in school. She encouraged her children to participate in sports and most of all to enjoy life. Alice said, "My father, on the other hand was somewhat of a grouch and a sourpuss, loved to gamble, take in Western movies, and eat out when we could afford it." He had good carpentry skills and always built his family a Japanese bathhouse where ever the family lived.

The happy life of the Noguchi family came to an abrupt end when President Roosevelt signed Executive Order 9066. In April of 1942, they were ordered to leave their home and way of life and were sent to the Turlock Assembly Center, a converted racetrack in California. The horse stalls accommodated a minimum of five people. The Noguchi family felt lucky in one sense, as the Army had run out of horse stalls when they arrived. Instead their abode was a single room in a crude, hastily constructed barrack.

Alice said, "This was a shocking and frightening experience after a lifetime of freedom. The camp was surrounded by barbed wire fence with armed guards in the watch towers. It was difficult for my parents to adjust, but we youngsters soon made friends and made the most of it." Alice learned to jitterbug at the dance classes and enjoyed the songfests. For Alice, going to church in the outdoors instead of the stuffy church was inspirational.

The Noguchis were at the Turlock Assembly Center for approximately five months, until they were moved under armed guard to the Gila River Relocation Center in the Arizona desert on the Gila River Indian Reservation. There were two camps, the Canal Camp and the Butte Camp, located about three miles apart. The total number of internees was 15,000 for the combined camps. Each tar-paper barrack had four rooms with four to six people per room. There were fourteen barracks to a block, a latrine and shower, a laundry room, and a large mess hall. Each block had an Issei block manager who was more or less a figurehead.

Each camp had a hospital staffed by available physicians, registered nurses, and auxiliary help. With limited equipment and skilled personnel, death during surgery or from a serious illness was not uncommon. There was a fire department, security forces, a post office, and various administration buildings. Schools were quickly established from kindergarten through the twelfth grade. The schools were credentialed and staffed by teachers who were volunteers from the outside or from qualified teachers within the camp. The high school curriculum was limited compared to outside schools but adequate for college preparation. School activities included sports, band, chorus, and special clubs.

Alice remembered:

> As a teenager in the junior and senior years I did not realize the dedication and sacrifice involved in these Caucasian teachers who volunteered to come to these desolate areas to teach a group of students, a group of people whom they knew so little about, as few Japanese people lived in Arizona or other states where the relocation camps were built.

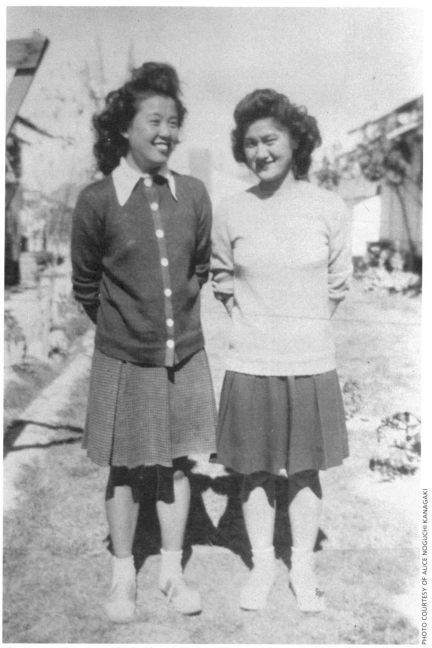

Teenagers, Alice Noguchi (left) and Corky Histatom interned at Butte Camp, Gila River Relocation Center in Arizona (1944).

These volunteer teachers were surprised to find that the Japanese American students were bright and eager to learn and presented very few disciplinary problems. These teachers in turn provided the encouragement and support for the students to perform to the best of their abilities and to continue on to higher education. The percentage of students going on to college from these camps was higher than the national average.

For the Issei parents, these were bleak years of apprehension and fear for the outcome of the family's future and for dwindling finances. Wages in camp amounted to less than a dollar a day. Alice's father was a mess hall supervisor and he received $19 a month. Her mother was a kitchen helper earning $16. There was a loss of family unity as the older children ate their meals with their friends rather than with their parents and because they were rarely home together in their one room, except at night to sleep.

Leisure activities were plentiful; there were competitive team sports, dances on the weekend, a library, and for the ladies, sewing and English classes. Women took an interest in their appearance, and the beauty parlor was active. Alice said, "Mother, who always wore her hair in a bun, got a permanent, much to my father's annoyance."

Gila River Relocation Center had a surprise visit from Eleanor Roosevelt. Alice recalls, "Mrs. Roosevelt made a special visit to our high school, and her picture appears in our high school annual. She re-established the fact that she cared about us."

Among the internees were many experienced produce growers who tapped into the canal water and turned the desert wasteland into lush produce farms, supplying the kitchens with fresh vegetables and marvelous melons of all sorts. Some of the other camps received melons from Gila River. There were pig farms to utilize the kitchen garbage, chickens, and some cattle. Camouflage netting was made at Gila River, providing more jobs for the evacuees. Alice said, "We were situated on the reservation grounds of the Gila River Indian community, home of the Pima and Maricopa tribes, and there were frequent visits from the Native Americans. The Indians came riding in buckboards and

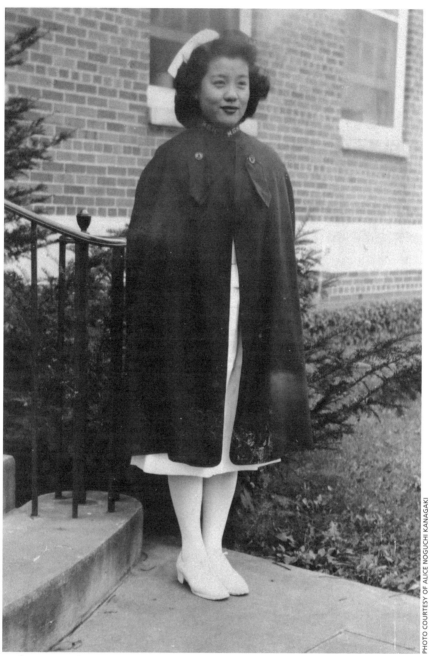

Cadet Nurse Alice Noguchi at Madison General Hospital School of Nursing, Madison, Wisconsin (1945).

on horseback to view us with much curiosity. Later friendships were formed and some sports competitions ensued."

Alice had been inspired by an older sister of a friend, a registered nurse who worked in the camp hospital. She saw her going to work one day, all in white from cap to shoes and wearing a navy blue nurse's cape, looking like a poster model. Alice was determined to someday be a nurse. Her father objected and told Alice that a person as scatterbrained as she and a tomboy by nature would embarrass the family with her failure. After Alice's mother intervened, her father relented.

During the final months of Alice's senior year of high school, plans for her future were bleak. Then her cousin wrote and told her that she was enrolled in a school of nursing in Madison, Wisconsin, and had joined the U.S. Cadet Nurse Corps. The cousin suggested that Alice consider this route. Alice jumped at the chance and although a late applicant, she was accepted. Alice said that her cousin was a model student and that the director must have assumed that she would be equally competent. Alice added that she and her cousin were as different as night and day. The kind director told her to work hard and she would do fine. Alice left for new horizons shortly after her high school graduation of June 1944, two years and a few months after her family's arrival.

Alice successfully completed the arduous three-year program, became a registered nurse, and worked for nearly 40 years and now retired plays golf almost every day. Alice is grateful for the education she received through the Corps. Otherwise, she would not have been able to afford her nursing education. Alice said that had she been asked or expected to enter the armed services upon completion of her program, she would have been proud to serve. Her three brothers all served in the military during World War II, and her joining would have been a natural progression.

Alice adds, "I was proud of the fact that my brothers were in the service as the general attitude was to prove to all that we were indeed loyal and worthy citizens, and why not, after all: we were born in the United States, we were citizens and knew no other country or culture."

7 Health Care in Camp

収容所の健康管理

URING THE FIRST YEAR of internment, the building of the hospitals was behind schedule; some were not completed until the end of 1942. There was also a shortage of equipment, many supplies, and medicines. The biggest problem of all was too few medical and nursing personnel. The result was overworked doctors and nurses and delays in treatment.[1] Yoshiye Toasaki, a Japanese physician from San Francisco, California, went early to California'a Manzanar Relocation Center to prepare for the incoming evacuees. His story appears in the 1982 government report of the Commission on Wartime Relocation and Internment of Civilians. Part of it follows:

> Equipment sent in for the medical care was the usual packaged unit for a military emergency hospital. To obtain necessary supplies such as vaccines for children, laboratory materials for tests, and special medication for pregnant women, I had to depend on generous contributions of a few friends until the government could set up its usual channels. Problems of formula preparation, since barracks had no water, no stove, only a single electric light in the center of a room created much hardship for the mothers who had to care for newborn infants and children… In due time the Military Emergency Hospital Unit (equipment) arrived as

did medical staff among the evacuees. For me, it was a matter of 14-16 hours per day of struggle and frustration.[2]

Health care providers were shaped by gender, racial, and medical hierarchies. Each camp employed a male Caucasian medical director who supervised the Japanese American doctors. The well-paid Caucasian registered nurses, regardless of experience, supervised the Nisei registered nurses and trained the nurse aides. The WRA hospital and health care system needed the labor of the internees, but the authority was kept in the hands of the white workers.[3]

When camp officials began recruiting women to train as nurse aides, they wanted Nisei women. Issei women were neglected not only because of their citizenship but because of their difficulties with the English language as well as their lack of healthcare training and expertise. Nearly seventy Issei women listed their occupation to be midwifery, yet none were ever employed as childbirth attendants within the camps. Before the war most Issei women gave birth at home attended by a Japanese midwife. Their practice flourished among members of the immigrant generation who had their babies between 1910 and 1940. Like some European immigrant midwives, Issei midwives often received their training in midwifery school in their native country.[4]

The training of high school students and other interested evacuees for nurse aide and orderly work was critical in solving the War Relocation Authority's (WRA's) nurse shortage. The 150 hour course covered taking temperatures, giving bed baths and enemas, and making beds. Instruction included the protocol for nurse aides and student nurses of that day: Keep busy; there is always cleaning to be done. Don't talk with the patients or sit on their beds. Stand up in the presence of doctors, and supervising and graduate nurses.[5]

Nurse aides assisted new mothers in the care of their newborn babies, and student nurses staffed the delivery rooms. Nearly 6,000 babies were born in the relocation camps during the internment years.[6] At Heart Mountain in Wyoming, visitors to the maternity ward were

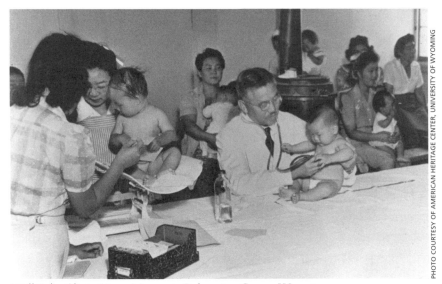

Well Baby Clinic, Heart Mountain Relocation Center, Wyoming.

banned initially. Later the husbands were allowed the privilege of visiting their wives and newborn children in the evening. Studies for that camp show that most mothers breast-fed their babies. A community-wide formula and milk distribution was established for formula-fed infants but was abandoned in the summer of 1943 before the oncoming fly season, as refrigeration was not available. Susan McKay reports in her study that the infant mortality rate at Heart Mountain was probably better than both state and national rates for that time.[7]

Health care, according to government records, was the centerpiece of public welfare provision at the WRA centers. Here many Japanese Americans, especially from the rural areas, received more health care than they had ever received before. Camp health care services mirrored those developed by the U.S. military forces, which equaled or exceeded those available to the average American during the World War II era.[8]

Health care authorities reported that camp hospitals could not run without the assistance of the nurse aides. In fact the nurse aides provided most of the nursing care, with the graduate nurses acting as supervisors. Nurse aides outnumbered the rest of the nursing staff.

For example, in 1944 at Poston, Arizona (the largest and the hottest of the camps), seventy-five Nisei nurse aides provided the nursing care of patients with supervision from fourteen graduate nurses—five white, five black, and four Issei.[9]

As a result of nationwide medical personnel shortages, some administrative physicians employed by the government were not the best. The Japanese American evacuee physicians were often better educated and more current in medical practice than their Caucasian supervisors. At Manzanar, a Caucasian doctor set limits on work by the evacuee doctors in charge of the ward, limiting the efficiency of the medical program. At Tule Lake in California, the elderly physician in charge was not aware of and would not allow newer medical procedures. After a great deal of protest from evacuees, he departed.[10] One Nisei nurse aide from Topaz in Utah tells this story:

> I was president of the nurse aides, and we were asked to join the medical staff to strike against the administration. Our medical staff consisted of Japanese evacuee physicians. The grounds for the strike was that our doctors could not prescribe oxygen and other special treatments for our patients. After much discussion, we finally agreed. I was working the Communicable Disease Unit on the p.m. shift, and the strike was scheduled to begin at midnight. The patients were frightened and we agreed to go back to the unit until the night shift came on. The strike was over by 3 a.m.[11]

The Japanese American evacuee physicians were not striking over wages. Even though they only received $19 a month for their long hours of work their concern was their patients.

The WRA asserted that the evacuees' physical health remained satisfactory. A 1946 comparison of death rates in the camps to deaths in the U.S. population as a whole found lower death rates in the former. But statistics don't tell the whole story. Children with mental retardation could not be cared for in camps. Tuberculosis and other serious illnesses, such as mental breakdowns, meant the removal of these evacuees with special problems to state institutions.[12]

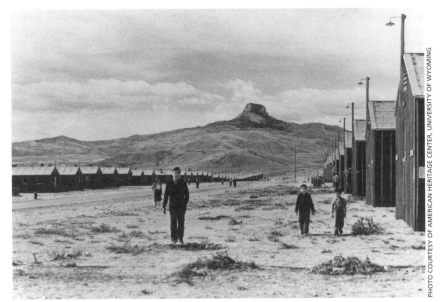

Barracks covered with tar paper at Heart Mountain, Wyoming housed 12,000 evacuees. The camp was named after the peak in the background.

Tuberculosis was the third leading cause of death in the camps, accounting for 206 deaths. The disease held a "quiet legacy" and because of the stigma attached, internees hesitated to seek treatment for fear of social ostracism. It was difficult to find volunteers to work as nurse aides in the tuberculosis wards.[13] One Nisei woman reported that she was a nurse aide and had worked on the communicable disease ward in spite of the fact that she had a positive skin test. Then she had an opportunity to leave camp and attend a school of nursing. She became sick on her travel to enter the school and was found to have a full-blown case of tuberculosis.[14]

Lives began and others ended in the relocation camps. The Public Health records for the Granada Relocation Center in Colorado show 300 births and 89 deaths for the three year internment period. Today, a few graves mark the spot where 8,000 people of Japanese ancestry were once interned behind barbed wire. In all the centers, the majority of families of the deceased chose to have their loved ones' remains cremated. The ashes were stored in the WRA storehouse awaiting the time when families could take the remains of their loved ones home for internment.[15]

With families confined to barracks and 250 people sharing the washing, laundry, and bathing facilities, small wonder that communicable diseases such as measles, pertussis, scarlet fever, chicken pox, tuberculosis, and impetigo were rampant. Public Health Records for Granada show a startling number of communicable diseases during the first year of evacuation. Due to the overcrowded populace, children contracted childhood diseases in great numbers. Problems with improper food handling accounted for the 53 evacuees who became ill from food poisoning during the month of January 1943.[16] These diseases could have been better controlled had hand-washing facilities been more available.

Varicella or chicken pox had the highest number of incidences (117) during the first year of internment at Granada. Children can become

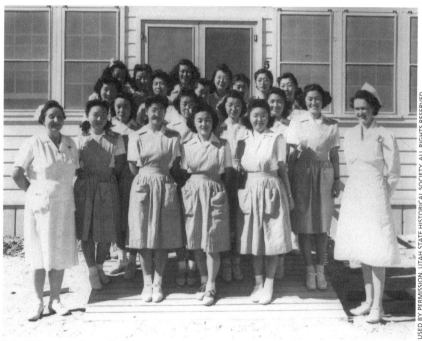

Nisei Nurse Aides with supervisors.

very sick and miserable from the pox and also have complications of lifelong consequence. In 1942, the State of Colorado did not require quarantine for chicken pox, but the public health officer took extra precautions and confined all children with pertussis to their "homes."[17]

On November 1, 1942, a Japanese registered nurse was assigned school nurse duties at Granada. One of her tasks was to check students with a communicable disease before the children could return to school. In December she checked 264 students for readmission.[18] The Army style barracks allotted each family, regardless of size, one room. It is hard to imagine how families cared for sick children with water, bathing, and latrine facilities blocks away and with the communal eating arrangements.

As evacuees built up immunity and environmental health protection improved, the second and third years at Granada showed a remarkable decrease in incidences of childhood communicable diseases. Pneumonia, both lobar and bronchia, showed an increase during the second year. This disease, which is more prevalent among adults and seniors, may indicate a factor of stress that lowers resistance to disease.

Dust was a major problem at most of the camps. In the spring of 1943, a Granada health care worker complained that dust arising at the camp during periods of moderate and high winds was a health hazard. In 1944, again a report was issued stating that the residents experienced dust storms three or four times a month for eight months out of the year. The only adequate protection from the dust storms was the planting of vegetation, but the water shortage was acute and there was no way to solve the problem.[19] Today the area remains dry and desolate.

It was clear that the detainees themselves provided most of the health care, with no representative voice in management or administration. Without their volunteer services, the WRA health care system would have been a disaster. Evacuee student nurses filled vital positions beyond their past training. Suzu Shimizu Kunitani, whose story follows, said, "I was assigned floor nurse duties in the Manzanar Hospital

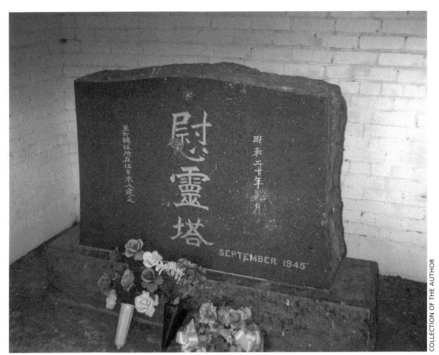

Grave site at the former Granada Relocation Center in Colorado.

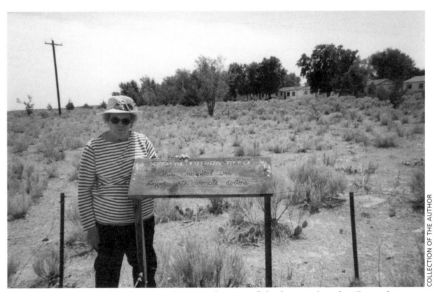

Return to sagebrush. Author standing on the site of the hospital at the Granada Relocation Center in Colorado. Granada had a population of 12,000.

with only eight months of basic nursing at the University of California. I struggled through that experience as best as I knew how."

Despite the hardships and restrictions of camp life, Japanese Americans used their pivotal role in the camp health care system to benefit the camp residents. They turned confinement into an opportunity to provide as much free health care as possible for their people.[20]

Life in the relocation centers under the WRA continued to be regimented and meant waiting not just for food and facilities, but also to see what would happen next. To prepare for the future seemed futile. Mitsu Hasegawa Nakada, whose story also follows, had been a student nurse for nine months at the Los Angeles County Hospital School of Nursing when Pearl Harbor was bombed. At the Heart Mountain Relocation Center in Wyoming, she served as head nurse on the surgical ward. She said, "We weren't abused. We had adequate food and we all worked. The hardest part was not knowing how long we would be there."[21]

Notes and References

[1] Report of the Commission on War Time Relocation of Internment of Civilians, *Personal Justice Denied*, (Washington, D.C.: GPO, 1982):163-4.

[2] Report, 143-4.

[3] Ibid.

[4] Susan L. Smith, "Women Health Workers and the Color Line in the Japanese 'Relocation Centers' of World War II," *Bulletin of the History of Medicine*, 73, no. 4, (Winter 1999):597.

[5] Inventory of Japanese American Evacuation and Resettlement Records: (1942-1946), Granada Public Health Reports from October 1942 through November 1945. The Bancroft Library Collection Number BANC MSS 6714c. (Berkeley, California: University of California).

[6] Smith, 599.

[7] Susan McKay, "Maternal Health Care at a Japanese American Relocation Camp, 1942-1945: A Historical Study," *Birth*, 24, no. 3, (September 1997):192.

[8] Smith, 588.

[9] Smith, 595.

[10] Report, 164.

[11] Anonymous, Nisei Cadet Nurse Project, Boulder, Colorado, 15 May 1999.

[12] Report, 164.

[13] Gwenn M. Jensen, "System Failure: Healthcare Deficiencies in the World War II Japanese American Detention Centers," *Bulletin of the History of Medicine*, 73, no. 4, (Winter 1999):621.

[14] Anonymous, Nisei Cadet Nurse Project, Boulder, Colorado, 3 March 2002.

[15] *Inventory of the Japanese American Evacuation and Resettlement Records.* (Microfilms, 1942-1946 Collection Number: BANC MSS 67/14C. Box Numbers 301 & 302.)

[16] Ibid.

[17] Ibid.

[18] Ibid.

[19] Jensen, 612.

[20] Jensen, 624.

[21] Mitsu Hasegawa Nakada, interview by author, Homer, Alaska: 28 April 1995.

Suzu Shimizu Kunitani

Life came to a halt with a possible doomed future.

SUZU SHIMIZU KUNITANI was following her parents desire that she pursue a college education, and she decided that a nursing career would be a likely profession. Her older brother was enrolled in medical school, which influenced her decision to choose nursing. Suzu was born and raised in a rural area in Centerville, California. Her parents were fruit farmers. They raised their children to be loyal and conscientious U.S. citizens and encouraged them to get good grades and to be model students. Suzu's parents worked long hours, seven days a week and provided their children with a healthy, caring environment. The family participated in Japanese community activities such as picnics, movies, and school programs. The children attended Japanese school classes after their regular schooling.

Suzu was enrolled in the University of California School of Nursing and approximately eight months into her training when she and those of Japanese descent were ordered to leave the West Coast. She went home to help her mother and three younger siblings pack up and leave their home, schools, and work. Her father's demise was in 1940. Suzu's mother stored all of the farm equipment and furniture in a neighbor's shed for the duration of the internment. (Those items mostly disappeared and were no longer there when the family returned in 1946.) The family was bused to Tanforan, an assembly center in south San Francisco that had been a racetrack. The smaller families were assigned to horse stalls, which contained remnants of the former occupants. Suzu said, "For me the Tanforan experience was traumatic and bewildering. Life came to a halt with a possible doomed future."

After three to four months, the families were shipped to Manzanar Relocation Center in the middle of the night by train. It was another frightening experience as the shades were drawn and the military police were in charge. Manzanar was located at the base of Mount Whitney, a desert-like remote area in southeastern California. The Shimizus were housed in crudely built barracks with no inner walls. There was one small window and cracks in the walls and flooring that allowed the cold and dust to blow in. In summers, the evacuees suffered from the dust storms and heat. In the winter, they were unaccustomed to the freezing cold.

Suzu said, "I was assigned floor nurse in the Manzanar Hospital with only eight months of basic nursing at the University of California Hospital. I struggled through that experience as best I knew how." One bright spot at Manzanar was that she met her future husband, Kazuo Kunitani. Suzu learned that she could leave camp providing she had a plan for relocation. She began writing to schools of nursing and discovered that the University of Colorado School of Nursing was admitting Japanese American students. In the 1940s only ten per cent of the schools of nursing offered a bachelor degree of science. At the University of Colorado, Suzu could complete her degree program. The other added feature was the U.S. Cadet Nurse Corps, which paid tuition, board, room, uniforms, and a small stipend.

The war effort stretched nursing resources, and there was pressure to shorten nursing courses. Henrietta Loughran, Director of the CU School of Nursing, found a way for the school to participate in the Corps and at the same time to maintain degree status for the students enrolled in the university. Mrs. Loughran was distressed by the relocation of West Coast Japanese American to camps in Western states. She collaborated with directors of university schools in Washington and California for the direct transfer of Japanese American students from the West Coast.[1] Suzu was one of more than a dozen nursing students who would benefit.

The University of Colorado School of Nursing was progressive in other ways. Zipporah Parks Hammond, the first Black student to be admitted into the university program was Suzu's classmate. Suzu and Zipporah, with interracial bonds, maintain a close friendship to this day.

While the training was rigorous, with long hours, Suzu never regretted her experience and felt that her education had given her a good foundation for her nursing career. The administration, the staff, and her classmates were friendly, considerate, and accepting. Suzu graduated in March of 1946 and she later recollected, "The Cadet Nurse Corps restored some of my faith and trust in the U.S. government. I suppose if the war had continued and the government had wanted me to serve in the armed forces, I would have been willing to do so. As it was, the war had ended and I went back to California to help my mother and siblings resettle in Northern California."

Suzu married her Manzanar sweetheart, an Army veteran, and together they raised four children in their home town of Centerville, California. When her children became school age, Suzu worked as a public health nurse. After 50 years, Suzu revisited her alma mater, the University of Colorado School of Nursing in Denver, Colorado. She said, "I was amazed at the growth and advancement in the school program. I enjoyed seeing the history and the pictures of all the graduating classes on the walls. It brought back good memories. I loved revisiting with a handful of old classmates."

Mitsu Hasegawa Nakada

*We were frightened as we had been told people might try to
kill us because we were Japanese, but we were safe wearing
our cadet nurse uniforms.*

WORLD WAR II WAS gaining momentum. On May 12, 1942, with tears
streaming down her face, a student nurse from the Los Angeles General
Hospital School of Nursing peered through the fence surrounding the
Hollywood Presbyterian Church. She had come to say goodbye to her
classmate and Japanese American friend, Mitsu Hasegawa. The friend
said, "But you are like us and we are like you," as Mitsu boarded the bus
for the Pomona Army Assembly Center in California.

Two weeks before, Japanese American employees of the Los Angeles
General Hospital had assembled in the auditorium to receive their
orders for relocation somewhere in the Midwest. The group, including doctors, nurses, pharmacists, secretaries, and student nurses, were
given two weeks to get ready for the move. Mitsu was completing nine
months as a student nurse with the Los Angeles General Hospital
School of Nursing and recalls how hard it was to plan as they didn't
know where they were going. She guessed that they would be going to
the desert and made culottes, but sewed both legs together and couldn't
get into them.

The Pomona Fairgrounds had been hastily converted to an assembly
center to receive the Japanese evacuees. After her arrival, Mitsu stood in
line waiting to receive her family's barrack number. She was pulled out
and asked if she would be in charge of making formula for the babies at
the center. Mitsu had never used a coal/wood stove before but managed
to make a fire and boil water for the babies' formula.

Three months later Mitsu again boarded a bus that took her to the railroad station where she and her group boarded a train for an unknown destination. Mitsu watched a lady being loaded on a stretcher through the window of a passenger train car. Stifled and hot, they rode for several days and nights with the blinds pulled down. Then permission was given to raise the shades for a brief time. The train was winding through a steep mountain canyon, and later the evacuees learned that they were passing through the Colorado Rockies.

The first group of Japanese American evacuees from the Pomona Assembly Center arrived at the Heart Mountain Relocation Center near Cody, Wyoming, on August 12, 1942. Mitsu said, "Because I had nine months of experience as a student nurse, I was given the assignment of charge nurse on the surgical unit. Mrs. Ginzo Nakada, the lady with paralysis whom I had seen being loaded onto the train was now my patient." The patient and nurse soon learned that their families had attended the same Japanese Holiness Church in Los Angeles. Mitsu remembered the family arriving at the church in a Hupmobile, a luxury car of the thirties, and their twelve kids piling out of the car to attend Sunday School.

Mrs. Nakada was scheduled for surgery. Her son Henry Nakada, who was training at Camp Shelby, Mississippi, with the Japanese American 442 Regimental Combat Team, was granted a furlough to give blood for his mother's pending surgery. Henry said that he was shocked when he visited his family at Heart Mountain Relocation Center. When he got off the bus he walked past the military police barracks to get to the ten-strand barbed wire fence with more strands at the top and machine gun emplacements along the fence.

Henry didn't have a chance to get acquainted with Mitsu on his leave, but his mother asked him to do something nice for the nurses for the good nursing care she was receiving at the camp hospital. Henry sent a big box of chocolates, a rare treat for the interned nurses. As charge nurse, Mitsu thought it her duty to write Henry a thank you note. Henry Nakada, who would soon be deployed to the war front in Europe, answered and asked Mitsu to write to him. Mitsu wasn't sure what to write and asked her Nisei friends to join her in writing to Henry. The letters from the cadet nurses would occasionally catch up with Henry as he moved with the battlefronts in Italy and France. Those letters were a great morale booster for the soldier who helped rescue the Lost Battalion and was the recipient of three Purple Hearts.

Mitsu had worked one year at Heart Mountain Relocation Hospital when she learned about the U.S. Cadet Nurse Corps. With family resources tied up, here was an opportunity to finish her nursing education and to do something for her country. She submitted her request to the Relocation Board, and they granted her release if she could find a school of nursing that would accept her. She first went to Elgin, Illinois and found a job working in a home for orthopedic impaired children. Here she began her search for a school of nursing and discovered the Protestant Episcopal Hospital School of Nursing in Philadelphia, Pennsylvania. Mitsu's application was accepted, and the school gave her six months credit for her previous work. This school of nursing was one of two in the state of Pennsylvania accepting Japanese American student nurses in 1943.

When in the Cadet Nurse Corps, Mitsu remembers a time when she joined four Japanese American cadet nurses on a trip to Florida. She said, "We were often frightened as we had been told people might try to kill us because we were Japanese, but we were safe wearing our cadet nurse uniforms." Protestant Episcopal was a large hospital with 5,000 patients, and Mitsu had two and one half years to finish the course. Because of her extensive past experiences, the school deliberated as to her placement. As a senior cadet nurse, Mitsu was assigned charge nurse duty for the medical pediatrics ward.

When the war ended, Henry Nakada was one of the first soldiers to be discharged. Wounded three times, he had missed very little combat, but near the end of the war he began to feel that he would not get out alive. Henry said that he started living a day at a time, which had made a great difference in his life. Henry's brother George served with the same unit and was killed in action in Italy. The record for the most sons in military service to serve in World War II goes to Mr. and Mrs. Ginzo Nakada. The Nakadas, evacuated from Long Beach, California, and interned at Heart Mountain, gave nine sons in the fight for freedom.[2]

Back in America, Henry's first stop was to visit Mitsu and her friends. He immediately fell in love with Mitsu and asked her to marry him. Henry was surprised when Mitsu said "yes" but she wanted to get her parents' permission. Mitsu's father came from a Samurai family, and both sides of her family had crests sufficiently high in Japanese society. Mitsu's first cousin married into the Emperor's family. The Hasegawas were now relocated in Pennsylvania, and Henry and Mitsu paid them a visit. Mitsu's parents suggested that they wait three months and if they still wanted to get married they would give them their blessing.

Another hurdle faced Mitsu, as student nurses could not marry and remain in school during the 1940s. One of the student nurses married in secret, was found out, and ousted. Mitsu made an appointment with Director of Nursing Doris Mathes. She saw that times were changing and gave Mitsu permission to marry. The couple was married on December 22, 1945, at the Episcopal Chapel, and both Nisei and Caucasian friends took part in the wedding. Mitsu was fortunate in finding a nurse administrator willing to risk going beyond traditional practice for that day; first, to admit Japanese American women into her school of nursing, and second, to break down another barrier in allowing women to marry and continue their nursing education.

Mitsu and Henry Nakada raised three boys. Mitsu specialized in pediatric nursing and public health. Henry became a professor of biochemistry and spent two years in Japan as the Director of the University of California Tokyo Study Center located at the International Christian University. The Nakadas learned about the culture of their ancestry and picked up some Japanese language they had forgotten. Mitsu visited her family in Tokyo.

After Henry's retirement from academia, Mitsu and Henry moved to Homer, Alaska. Mitsu ended her nursing career as an itinerant school nurse in bush communities. Mitsu was also an artist and made fish prints using a traditional Japanese method. She crocheted, knitted, and kept a lovely garden. Clamming, fishing, and being out-of-doors on Kachemak Bay were high on her list as to how to spend a perfect day.[3]

References and Notes

[1] Diane B. Hamilton, *Becoming a Presence Within Nursing: The History of University of Colorado School of Nursing, 1898-1998*, (Denver, Colorado: The University of Colorado School of Nursing, 1999):54-7.

[2] Bill Hosokawa, *Nisei: The Quiet Americans*. (New York: William Morrow and Company, Inc., 1969):419. The Nakada nine sons in service included: Yoshinao, with the Office of Strategic Services; Henry and George with the 442nd; John with military intelligence in Alaska; Saburo, Masoru, James, and Yoshio with military intelligence in the Pacific; and Stephen with the Japanese language school.

[3] "Mitsu Hitsu Hasegawa Nakada," Obituaries, *Homer News*, died 7 October 2001 at the age of 81. Her family said that above all, "Mitsu collected friends."

8 From Camp to the Corps

牧
容
所
より
看護
部隊
に

Some 3,500 Japanese American students in the three Pacific Coast states were among those ordered to leave their colleges, universities, and schools of nursing under Executive Order 9066. In early May of 1942, Milton S. Eisenhower, director of the newly organized War Relocation Authority (WRA), telephoned Clarence Pickett. He asked the prominent Quaker leader to call together various groups to work on the problem of student relocation and to organize a national council to carry out the program. Picket agreed to take on the task.[1]

Governor Culbert Olson of California, also concerned about the student problem, wrote to President Franklin Roosevelt. In his letter Olson explained that the evacuation had interrupted the education of many loyal Japanese American young people. The President took note and replied:

> I am deeply concerned that the American-born Japanese college stu-
> dents shall be impressed with the ability of the American people
> to distinguish between enemy aliens and staunch supporters of the
> American system.[2]

Roosevelt approached Eisenhower about the Japanese American student problem, and he was relieved to know that progress was taking place. In his book, *The President is Calling*, Eisenhower said that if the President had better understood the human problem he might not have ordered the mass evacuation.[3]

In March of 1942, Margaret Tracy, Director of the University of California School of Nursing, expressed concern for her Japanese American students. She wrote Claribel Wheeler of the National League of Nursing Education for advice. She pointed out that she had 22 Japanese American students who were all scholastically at the top of their class. The nursing faculty found them to be above average, both in the classroom and on the wards. She posed this question: "Do you think there are schools of nursing in this country, east of the Sierras, which might accept these students as transfers?"[4]

A meeting of national nurse leaders was held a short time later, and Wheeler read Tracy's letter to the group. According to nurse historians, the nurse leaders were in agreement that under the circumstances they doubted if any school of nursing in the United States would be willing to take the Japanese American students. Professional nurses could take little credit for their indifferent handling of this sensitive problem.[5]

Margaret Tracy was far from consoled by the evasive response and was determined to do the best for her Nisei students. She found the solution for some of her students through Henrietta Adams Loughran, Director of the University of Colorado School of Nursing. In the early war years, Loughran, with support from Colorado Governor Ralph Carr, collaborated with the directors of the university schools of nursing in California and Washington, and made possible the direct transfer of students.[6]

One Japanese American student nurse enrolled in the Seattle College School of Nursing who benefitted from the Colorado program tells this story:[7]

> I did not go to a relocation center because Governor Carr of Colorado consented to take Japanese American students who were attending universities on the West Coast and I took the opportunity to transfer.

I left Seattle by train along with another Japanese American student nurse. No one of the Japanese race could go near the train depot so a handful of our Caucasian friends came to see us off. We slept in a single upper berth and the government paid our way. When I left, my parents were busy sorting out the things they could take to camp. I arrived in Denver in May of 1942 and was immediately enrolled in the University of Colorado School of Nursing.

A year later I had an opportunity to join the Cadet Nurse Corps. I wanted to join the war effort and my parents were not complaining about their incarceration in their letters. They were being taken care of and being fed. They wrote me that I should concentrate on my studies and not to worry about them. Without Governor Carr's brave and generous act, I would not have been able to finish my training as soon as I did. I was the only Nisei in my class but there were other Japanese Americans who were welcomed after me.

Throughout his political career Governor Carr demonstrated the courage to defend what he felt was right. Many Colorado historians believe this action cost Carr a seat in the United States Senate in the next election.[8] Carr never wavered on his stand and later made this statement:

If we do not extend humanity's kindness and understanding to these people, if we deny them the protection of the Bill of Rights, if we say they may be denied the privilege of living in any of the 48 states without hearing or charge of misconduct, then we are tearing down the whole American system.[9]

The National Japanese American Student Relocation was organized in Chicago on May 29, 1942. The membership included college presidents and deans, church leaders of all denominations and faiths, and the student YMCA and YWCA. The cost of operation was met through generous grants from church boards and philanthropic foundations. It was not until the end of 1942 that the government procedures for clearing colleges and students became sufficiently well organized to permit any great flow of students from camp to college.[10]

In 1943, the WRA began promoting the relocation of students, but there were obstacles to overcome. Financial means was the biggest hurdle, as families had been stripped of their monetary resources. Young people were also slow in leaving the centers because it was reported that repatriate groups were ridiculing the efforts of the loyal groups who wanted to make a place for themselves in the normal current of American life. Some parents were reluctant to see their families separated. Parents were especially cautious in the case of their daughters, whom they felt would be unprotected in the hostile world. The evacuees had lived a year in internment, and their morale was affected. They had been pushed around so much that they needed stability. They understood that internment at the camps would be for the duration of the war, and now the WRA expected them to make another difficult adjustment.[11]

Only a few students were fortunate in transferring to other educational institutions before the complicated red tape procedures went into effect. Finding a school of nursing that would accept Japanese American students continued to be a problem. Some nurse consultants advised schools of nursing not to accept Japanese American students. At a nursing conference in Lincoln, Nebraska, several directors of schools of nursing had received applications from Japanese Americans. They asked a visiting professor in nursing education her opinion on admitting these women. The professor took a pessimistic viewpoint, stating that there would always be mistrust in the minds of patients as well as the doctors and nurses. She stated that the students would be under FBI surveillance and advised against it.[12] Only one small Catholic school of nursing in Nebraska accepted Japanese American students. The St. Joseph's School of Nursing in the western part of the state admitted one student with Japanese ancestry in 1944 and a second in 1945.[13]

An American Journal of Nursing (AJN) editorial asked readers to consider the problem of the American girl of Japanese ancestry who was denied the right to enroll in a school of nursing or unable to complete a course that was interrupted when she was evacuated. A suggestion had been made that schools of nursing be established in relocation center hospitals. Nurse educators pointed out that the clinical resources in the relocation centers could not provide an adequate experience and education for student nurses.[14]

The nursing journal reported Nisei students who wished to enter schools of nursing encountered resistance not met by ordinary university students. Only 84 Japanese American women out of 371 had been able to finish their interrupted course in nursing, according to the AJN 1943 report. The editorial urged schools of nursing to take up the matter.[15] The editorial stated:

> It is the function of this magazine to place the facts before its readers and to urge careful, unbiased, and imaginative study of the situation by faculties of schools of nursing, members of hospital boards, and representative citizens, to the end that a solution may be found for loyal American girls whose ancestors happen to have been Japanese.[16]

During World War II, the nation faced one of the gravest nursing shortages in history. In spring of 1943, nurse training institutions and their associations, along with hospital groups, drafted a nurse training bill that would alleviate the shortage. In March of 1943, Representative Francis Bolton from Ohio introduced a bill "to provide for the training of nurses for the armed forces, governmental and civilian hospitals, health agencies and war."[17] A companion bill was introduced in the Senate with the provision that there would be no discrimination in the administration of the benefits and appropriations on account of race, creed, or color. Both houses unanimously passed the bill. The Nurse Training Act on June 15, 1943 was signed by the President and became public law.[18]

The nursing shortage would be alleviated through an extensive and accelerated program, the U.S. Cadet Nurse Corps, as the cadet nurses provided critical nursing services for the hospitals in which they trained. As senior cadet nurses, they would be available to serve in public health agencies, as well as veteran and military hospitals and other institutions where a shortage of nurses existed. The federal government paid the schools for tuition and fees for each student as well as maintenance for the first nine months of training. These funds enabled the schools to increase enrollments and to meet added costs.

As for the cadets, any young woman who could meet the admission requirements of an approved school of nursing participating in the program could join the U.S. Cadet Nurse Corps. The cadet would receive a complete scholarship and a monthly stipend as her personal allowance. In return the cadet signed a pledge to remain in essential nursing service, military or civilian, for the duration of the war.[19] For the Nisei young woman, interned in relocation camps, the Cadet Nurse Corps spelled freedom with an economic livelihood and education.

The Student Relocation Council, sponsored by the Friends Service Committee located in Philadelphia, worked tirelessly helping college-age Japanese Americans to relocate and to continue their education, dispelling myths and assuring administrators that loyal American citizens with Japanese ancestry made exceptional students. An advisory committee officer, Walter Godfrey, learned about the Cadet Nurse Corps and had questions for Dr. Thomas Parran, Surgeon General of the U.S. Department of Public Health Service. In his letter dated August 19, 1943, Godfrey wrote:

> It has been pointed out…that Negroes and Americans of Japanese ancestry are not eligible for such scholarships. I wonder if you could clear this matter up for me? It seems strange to me that there should be such a ruling when there has been no such order prohibiting them from joining such organizations as the WAAC (Women's Auxiliary Army Corps).[20]

Parran delegated Lucile Petry, director of the Cadet Nurse Corps, to respond and she sent Godfrey a copy of Public Law 74 of the 78th Congress, pointing out the introductory paragraph. It read, "There shall be no discrimination in the administration of the benefits and appropriations."[21] Here was a chance for Japanese American young women to join a uniformed service, to pursue an education, and to prove their loyalty.

Chairman of the Advisory Committee for Evacuees in Chicago, Rolland Schloerb, lost no time in sending dozens of schools of nursing the news that the Cadet Nurse Corps was open to Japanese American young women. Administrators of schools of nursing were assured that already the nurse students had proven their fine character, devoted attitude toward patients, scholarship, and loyalty. The concluding statement read, "In a war which we are fighting for democracy, we believe that it behooves all of us to weigh any action which might be interpreted as discriminatory."[22]

For the Nisei, the Student Relocation Council, sponsored by the Quakers in Philadelphia, will always be a symbol of the tolerance and democratic spirit of the American people. The WRA and private citizens also assisted Nisei young women in locating work on the outside and finding schools of nursing that would receive them.

Mae Hoshino Masuda's parents were farmers and lived in a rural area outside of Pendleton, Oregon. In December of 1941, Mae was working in a superintendent of schools' office and was fired when the war broke out. The family lived outside the military war zone so was not required to relocate. Mae's father had been a teacher in Japan and had many interests such as hunting, photography, and radio. Consequently, the Hoshinos had guns, cameras, and a short-wave radio, all of which were considered contraband and confiscated by the FBI.[23]

At this same time Mae was hospitalized with appendicitis, and she decided that she wanted to be a nurse. She spent the next three years submitting applications to schools of nursing, only to be rejected because patients and medical staff were ambivalent. She saw a Cadet Nurse Corps poster in a local store and was all the more determined to find a school of nursing that would accept her. She decided to go through the WRA Office at Minidoka, Idaho. Through this effort she was accepted into the Mother Cabrini Hospital School of Nursing in Chicago. Mae and nine Nisei cadet nurses graduated from this school of nursing.

Mary Kubota found a school of nursing with assistance from a private citizen. At the time of evacuation Mary's family consisted of her parents, two sisters, and a brother. They lived on a farm near Odell, Oregon and participated in local church activities and the Japanese American Citizen League (JACL). She and her family learned about the evacuation order when notices were posted on the utility poles.[24]

Mary and her family spent three months at the Puyallup Assembly Center in California and were then sent to the Minidoka Relocation Center in Idaho. Mary worked as a nurse aide at the hospital. One day a senator's daughter who lived nearby the camp came looking for a maid. She was a friend of the Minidoka camp director and hired Mary shortly after her interview. Part of Mary's time was spent in Washington, D.C., where she made a number of Nisei friends and learned about the Cadet Nurse Corps. Mary applied to the Bellevue School of Nursing in New York City, and her acceptance made her eligible to join the Corps.[25]

After receiving her nursing diploma from Bellevue, Mary continued her education and was inducted into the National Nursing Honor Society. Thanks to the Cadet Nurse Corps for her basic nurse education, Mary gave 38 years of nursing service, retiring as a director of nurses.

The stories of two other Nisei cadet nurses, Edith Yonemoto Ichiuji and Kaoru Morita Ehara, follow.

References and Notes

[1] Milton S. Eisenhower, *The President is Calling.* (Garden City, New York: Doubleday & Company, 1974):120.

[2] Ibid.

[3] Ibid, 121.

[4] Philip A. Kalisch and Beatrice J. Kalisch, *From Training to Education: The Impact of Federal Aid on Schools of Nursing in the U.S. During the 1940s,* (Vol. 1 of Final Report of NIH Grant NU 00443, December 1974):111-114.

[5] Ibid.

[6] Diane B. Hamilton, *Becoming a Presence Within Nursing: The History of the University of Colorado School of Nursing, 1898-1998.* (Denver, Colorado: The University of Colorado School of Nursing, 1999):56-7.

[7] Anonymous, Nisei Cadet Nurse Project, Boulder, Colorado, 1999.

[8] Bill Hosokawa, *Nisei: The Quiet Americans*, (New York: William Morrow and Company, Inc., 1969):225-6.

[9] "The Japanese in Our Midst" [Brochures from the Council of Churches, 1943]. Thomas Bodine Collection, Archives of Hoover Institution of War, Revolution and Peace, (Palo Alto, California).

[10] "From Camp to College" [Brochure, ca. 1942]. Thomas Bodine Collection, as in 9.

[11] "Preliminary Evaluation of the Resettlement Program at Jerome Relocation Center," [A report from the Project Analysis Series no. 5, 1943]. Thomas Bodine Collection, as in 9.

[12] Michele L. Fagan, "Nebraska Nursing Education during World War II," *Nebraska History*, (Fall, 1992):132.

[13] David Brueggemann, *The U.S. Cadet Nurse Corps: The Nebraska Experience*, Unpublished Masters Thesis, (Omaha: University of Nebraska, 1991).

[14] Editorial, "The Problem of Student Nurses of Japanese Ancestry," *American Journal of Nursing*, 10 (October 1943):895.

[15] Ibid.

[16] Ibid, 896.

[17] Federal Security Agency, *The U.S. Cadet Nurse Corps, 1943-1948*, (Public Health Service Publication No. 38, Washington, D.C.: Government Printing Office, 1950):15-20.

[18] Ibid.

[19] Ibid, 18-19 & 84.

[20] From the American Friends manuscript collection (ca. 1942-1945) (Seattle, Washington: University of Washington Library.) Letter to Dr. Thomas Parran, Surgeon General USPHS, 19 August 1943, from Walter Godfrey.

[21] Ibid. Letter to Walter Godfrey, 31 August 1943, from Lucile Petry, Director, Division of Nurse Education, USPHS.

[22] Ibid.

[23] Mae Hoshino Masuda, Nisei Cadet Nurse Project, Boulder, Colorado, 2001.

[24] Mary Kabota, Nisei Cadet Nurse Project, Boulder, Colorado, 1999.

[25] Ibid.

Yoshiko "Edith" Yonemoto Ichiuji

This was the highlight of my nursing career. I had come full circle.

YOSHIKO "EDITH" YONEMOTO ICHIUJI's parents worked hard on a small vegetable truck farm in a place called French Camp near Stockton, California. She and her siblings walked two miles each day to a small rural school and after school hours attended Japanese school. After graduation from high school, the happy-go-lucky young lady was enrolled in a pre-nursing degree program. Then came the devastating news of Pearl Harbor. Edith continued with her classes, finishing one semester and enrolling in the next semester. With the curfew on, Edith had to drop her evening chemistry class as the situation got worse, and she stopped attending classes mid-semester. Edith said, "All hopes of becoming a nurse were shattered."

On May 28, 1942, Edith's father's birthday, the six members of the Yonemoto family packed what they could carry and were taken to the Southern Pacific train station in Manteca, California, for parts unknown. With armed soldiers they traveled all night with shades drawn. Their destination? Manzanar Relocation Center in California, population 10,000. The party of almost 200 was the last group to arrive. Edith said it was scary. After filling their canvas bags with straw for their mattresses, the family of six settled down to share their one small room. Because they were the last to arrive, their group found little opportunity for work.

Edith went to the camp hospital and applied for nurse aide work and was hired. With no running water in the barrack hospital, the washing of hands was done in a basin filled with creosol-water solution. The strong disinfectant proved toxic to Edith's hands. After working there for six months, Edith developed a severe case of dermatitis. She then worked as a cashier at the co-op dry goods store, but the job held no challenge.

One day after a year in camp, Edith received a letter from the American Friends Service Committee, a Quaker group in Philadelphia, asking her if she would be interested in continuing her education. The letter, which she read over and over again, listed schools of nursing that had been cleared by the FBI and the WRA. The St. Mary's Hospital School of Nursing in Rochester, Minnesota, affiliated with the world famous Mayo Clinic was, on the list. Edith didn't know anyone in Minnesota or even know where it was. With the war on, her parents were reluctant to let her go.

Correspondence with the Quakers continued, encouraging Edith to pursue her nursing. Through them she learned about the U.S. Cadet Nurse Corps. Leaving camp was no easy task. After first dealing with the WRA and the FBI, she then had to be accepted by a school of

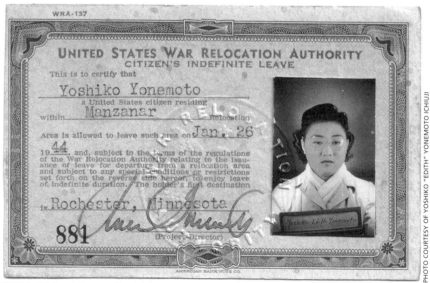

PHOTO COURTESY OF YOSHIKO "EDITH" YONEMOTO ICHIUJI

WRA Citizen's Leave Card. The war interrupted Yoshiko "Edith" Yonemoto Ichiuji's pre-nursing program. Two years would pass before she was granted leave from Manzanar to resume her nursing education.

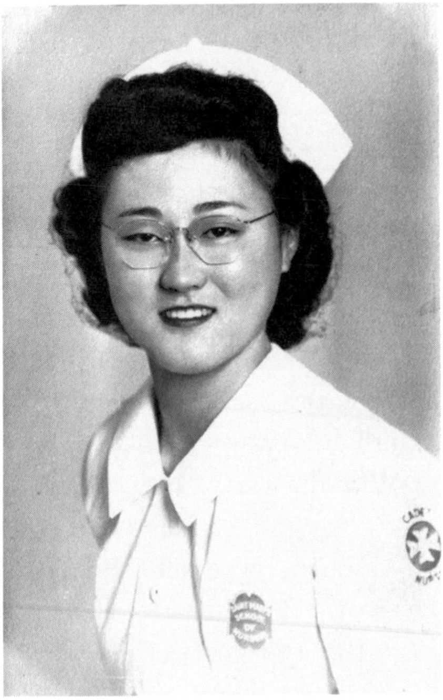

PHOTO COURTESY OF YOSHIKO "EDITH" YONEMOTO ICHIUJI

Edith Yonemoto Ichiuji, cadet nurse at St. Mary's Hospital School of Nursing in hospital uniform.

nursing. Edith ordered a foot locker from Sears and Roebuck. With her worldly possessions, she left Manzanar on a Greyhound bus. Edith said that she was "one scared twenty-year-old Nisei headed for St. Mary's Hospital School of Nursing."

Edith remembers the Franciscan sisters welcoming the Japanese American students and making them feel at home. Three years later Edith graduated and continued to work as a delivery room supervisor for two years. When her father died unexpectedly, she returned to French Camp to be with her family. Taking time out for marriage and raising three children, Edith resumed her nursing career as an obstetrical nurse. After more than thirty years of nursing service, Edith hung up her nursing cap and retired. Today her three children, inspired by their mother, carry on in health care professions: a daughter is an oncologist specialist, a son is a dentist, and another daughter is a pharmacist.

In 1998, Edith attended the JACL national convention in Philadelphia. The American Friends Service Committee sponsored a breakfast and there she had an opportunity to personally thank the committee for helping so many like herself whose education had been disrupted due to war hysteria and relocation. Edith said, "This was the highlight of my nursing career. I had come full circle."

Kaoru Morita Ehara

I am forever indebted to all these good people who helped two young inexperienced teenagers get a start on the outside.

KAORU MORITA EHARA grew up and attended schools in Oakland, California, and had decided that she would be a mathematics teacher. After the war broke out Kaoru and her family were evacuated to the Tanforan Assembly Center. They felt fortunate as they were placed in a newly constructed barrack instead of a horse stable. Kaoru was fifteen years of age and worked as a waitress during meal times.

In September 1942, all of the people from Tanforan Assembly Center were sent to the Topaz Relocation Center in Utah. Kaoru attended the camp high school and worked part time as a nurse aide in the Topaz hospital. She found this experience challenging and changed her career aspiration from teaching to nursing, much to the disappointment of her parents.

Kaoru had no financial means to go to nursing school. A mentor and a former church teacher contacted an acquaintance, Henry Toni, in St. Louis, Missouri. Henry researched the possibilities of Kaoru's relocating in St. Louis and the opportunities for schools of nursing. Kaoru, now a senior in high school, received an application for entering the St. Louis City Hospital School of Nursing along with a form for enrollment in the U.S. Cadet Nurse Corps.

In August 1944 Kaoru embarked on a train trip to St. Louis. Her civics teacher and supporter generously gave her and her friend, Bea, a twenty dollar bill and wished them well. "I am forever indebted to all these good people who helped two young inexperienced teenagers get a start on the outside," Kaoru said.

Upon arrival in St. Louis, Kaoru and her friend were met by Henry, who took them to his home. Both found housekeeping jobs for the interim before beginning their nursing education as cadet nurses at St. Lukes Hospital School of Nursing. With reflection Karou said, "Nursing provided me an honorable profession and I am happy that I was able to spend the next 40 years working as a registered nurse. So it is with gratitude, in spite of our incarceration, that I thank the United States government."

9 Nisei in the Corps

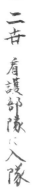

I N EARLY SUMMER OF 1944, the Student Relocation Council administrated by the American Friends Service Committee in Philadelphia was aware of apprehension in the relocation camps. Issei parents expressed concern in sending young people off to college in a world filled with prejudice. The Council enlisted the aid of various organizations in financing the return of a few Nisei who found acceptance in institutions of higher learning. College students returned to their former camps and met with high school graduates. They discussed relocation and college challenges with the new graduates and their parents. The returnees gave personal accounts of successful adjustment in the world outside. The students' presence lifted the morale of camp residents. Their work was commended by both evacuees and the relocation administration.[1]

Myths were dispelled regarding Caucasian nursing students ostracizing their Japanese American classmates. Elizabeth Lattell McQuale, a cadet nurse and roommate of a Nisei at the Protestant Episcopal Hospital School of Nursing in Philadelphia said:

> I left home a mousy little girl, but through my cadet nurse experience
> I became mature and outgoing. The biggest event of my life during
> those years of nurses training was getting to know another culture. My

Japanese American roommate, Jean Oda (now deceased), was a few years older and took me under her wing. Her college had been interrupted when she and her family were transported to Arizona to serve in a "concentration camp." From some of the tales she told me, it was not pleasant. Sand storms were frequent; infirmary facilities were meager. Sheets were hung to allow some privacy for patients.

Four Japanese American students were in my class of '46. I was constantly amazed how talented these American Japanese girls were. They could see a dress on a store model, copy the design, cut it out from newspaper for a pattern, then sew it up. "How did you do this?" I would ask. Always the reply, "My mother taught me."

Jean introduced me to classical music at the Academy of Music, light opera, open air summer music at Robin Hood Dell, and the live theater. Home-cooked Japanese food became part of my life so that even today I have maintained a curiosity for new foods from different cultures and countries and life all around me.[2]

The Protestant Episcopal Hospital School of Nursing in Philadelphia dated back to the days of the Civil War, but Dora Mathes, Director of the School of Nursing, was progressive for her time. Previous directors had been diploma graduates, but Dora had a master's degree and changes were in order. The student nurses appreciated not having to wear the formerly required black stockings and shoes, the bane of beginning nurse students dubbed "probies" (students on probation). Dora worked closely with the American Friends Service Committee. She was one of two directors of nursing schools in the mid-Atlantic states to first accept Japanese American student nurses during the early war years.

Rhoda Behrndt Kite, a graduate from Bellevue Hospital School of Nursing in New York City, sent this news clipping about her Japanese American classmate, Dorothy Kikuye Hayashi. The article read:

There were rocky detours in the road that Dorothy Kikuye Hayashi took to become a nurse, but the sweet-faced, spunky little Nisei kept right on going. Today she holds the coveted title at last. Yesterday (June 13, 1946) she received her bachelors degree and certificate of nursing from the Bellevue School of

Nursing at New York University. She was 1 of 11 of the 255 graduates to earn a degree. And she won the Bellevue Alumnae Award for both the highest scholarship average and excellence in nursing practice.[3]

The article continued to tell how winning the latter honor had taken Dorothy by surprise. Dorothy was quoted to say, "We all worked hard. During the war we were short of nurses and we all worked together." Then she quietly spoke of the obstacles that lay in her path. Dorothy was a second year nursing student at the University of California when the war came. She spent several months interned with her family in California and then at the Heart Mountain Relocation Center in Wyoming. She wanted to finish her nursing education and was able to get clearance from the camp. Dorothy went to Chicago and found that white collar jobs were unavailable for a Nisei. Finally she found work as a maid and saved every penny. Soon the formation of the U.S. Cadet Nurse Corps made it possible for Dorothy to resume her training. In December of 1943, after a year working as a housemaid, she enrolled in Bellevue, completing her degree in nursing in June of 1946.[4]

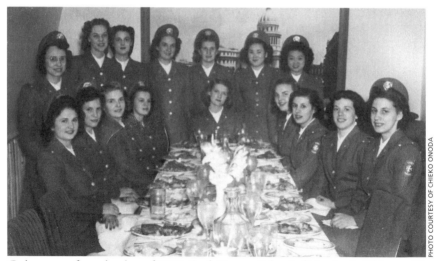

PHOTO COURTESY OF CHIEKO ONODA

Cadet nurses from the class of 1947, Cook County School of Nursing in Chicago. All U.S. Cadet Nurse Corps programs were fully integrated. Chieko Onoda (standing first on right) used nursing and linguistic skills in her future role as coordinator for the University of Illinois Global Health Program. She taught nurses in Chicago and Japan.

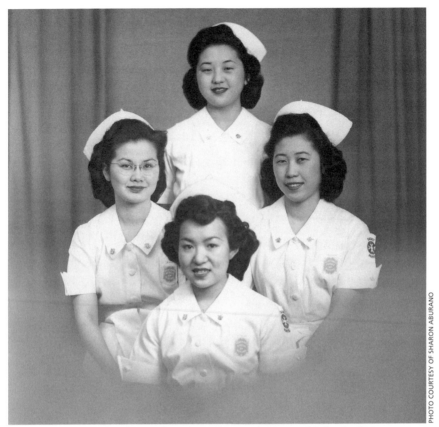

Cadet nurses in student hospital uniform, St. Mary's Hospital School of Nursing, Rochester, MN. Top: Mary (Izumi) Tamura. Middle: Left to right: Mary (Sagata) Tamura, Ida (Sakohira) Kawaguchi. Bottom: Sharon (Tanagi) Aburano.

Another Nisei cadet nurse said that she enjoyed fulfilling her dream to become a nurse and spent very little time thinking about the war and her family in camp. She was too busy working and learning and found no prejudice nor ill feeling concerning her race. She said, "Once, a patient asked me if I was French, probably because of my black hair. I smiled and passed the comment in silence, thinking to myself, 'This is the first time this lady has ever seen a Japanese American in this neck of the woods.'"[5]

Unlike other military segregated units, the U.S. Cadet Nurse Corps provided student nurses of Japanese ancestry an opportunity to serve with unquestionable integration in more than sixty hospitals and communities throughout the country during World War II. Records show that St. Mary's Hospital School of Nursing in Rochester, Minnesota, affiliated with the famous Mayo Clinic, admitted 42 Japanese American students, more than any other school of nursing in the country.[6]

In the 1940s most people east of the Mississippi had never seen a person of Japanese ancestry. This was a new experience for both the Nisei and the Americans. The Cadet Nurse Corps proved to be a boon for more than 350 Japanese American young women segregated and interned in relocation camps.[7] Like their soldier brothers, they wanted an opportunity to prove their loyalty and to serve their country in uniform. With courage and determination, they left their families behind barbed wire to face a hostile world and served their country as cadet nurses during World War II and early post-war years.

The stories of Sharon Tanagi Aburano, Ida Sakohira Kawaguchi, and Aiko Grace Obata Amemiya follow.

References and Notes

[1] Robert W. O'Brien, *The College Nisei*. (Palo Alto, California: Pacific Books, 1949): 68.

[2] Elizabeth Lattell McQuale, Nisei Cadet Nurse Project, Boulder, Colorado, 1995.

[3] From Rhoda Bemdt Kite, Nisei Cadet Nurse Story Project, Boulder, Colorado, 1994-1999. "Nisei Conquers Obstacles to Win Honors as Nurse," *New York World-Telegram*, 13 June 1946.

[4] Ibid.

[5] Anonymous, Nisei Cadet Nurse Project, Boulder, Colorado, 2001.

[6] Thelma Robinson, *Distribution of Nisei Cadet Nurses 1944-1946 by Region, States, City and Schools of Nursing*: (Unpublished data], Nisei Cadet Nurse Project, Boulder, Colorado, 2001.

[7] Ibid.

Sharon Tanagi Aburano

*The uniform stood for patriotism, and I was proud to show
that I was serving my country.*

SHARON TANAGI ABURANO, born in Seattle, Washington, was a
sophomore in high school when World War II broke out. The community in which she grew up was called the International District, and
her family ran a successful grocery store. The Tanagis' church affiliation
was Presbyterian, and Sharon was active in the teenage "Light Bearers"
group. World War II brought about the dissolution of a stable family
life and secure lifestyle for Sharon and her family. Eight weeks after
Pearl Harbor, Sharon's father, Koi Tanagi, along with many Japanese
community leaders, were suspect. Although no charges were ever filed
against him, Koi was imprisoned in Kooskia, Idaho, and two years
would pass before his family saw him again. Sharon's brother was serving at the Military Intelligence School in Minnesota.

Sharon and her mother's first detention was at the Puyallup
Assembly Center in Washington. The second move was four months
later to the Minidoka Relocation Center in Idaho. Sharon finished high
school in camp, worked part-time for the community service department, and served as a nurse aide. Sharon's mother knew she wanted to
go into nursing and realized that internment was for the duration of
the war, but no one knew how long that would be. Sharon's mother was
willing to let her go, but she wondered how she would find the financial
means since the family was stripped of all monetary resources. Sharon
said that she wanted to prove her patriotism as well as to acquire a
profession.

Father Tibesar, a Catholic priest who had followed his flock to the Minidoka Relocation Center in Idaho, gave Sharon information about the U.S. Cadet Nurse Corps. She wondered if she would be accepted into a school of nursing because of her ancestry. The Catholic Father suggested St. Mary's Hospital School of Nursing in Rochester, Minnesota, and he wrote the Franciscan sisters attesting to Sharon's moral character. Sharon said, "Father Tibesar advised me that my behavior would impact others who wished to leave camp. Therefore, I must endure any acts of prejudice and try to be a model student so it would be easier to place more interned students."

The next three years were spent studying and working for a diploma in nursing, and Sharon said the Franciscan nuns were wonderful teachers. The nurses' home, a spacious four story structure, housed 300 students and was connected to the hospital by a tunnel. Because Sharon had experience as a nurse aide, the basics like taking temperatures and blood pressures were easy for her. The cadet nurses' learning experiences were enriched with lectures from prominent visiting medical experts as well as the Mayo Clinic doctors. Extracurricular opportunities offered swimming, tennis, and on occasion a hike with fellow students to a local park for a picnic.

Sharon experienced a polio epidemic while she was in training. She cared for the patients in iron lungs (a respiration device) by putting their hands through the side holes for bathing and other care. She applied hot Kenny Packs for pain relief and cared for the critically ill patients. Sharon said the children dying from respiratory failure made her weep. One night there was a power outage, and the students off-duty rushed to the aid of their classmates who were working on the polio ward. When the electricity failed, the iron lungs operated manually. This was an exhausting and tense time for the staff on the polio ward and was terrifying for the patients. Enough volunteers were on hand when Sharon's group reached the tunnel so the Franciscan nuns gathered them in a circle to pray. They watched the darkened hospital and prayed that the emergency generators would come on. Miraculously no lives were lost.

Sharon enjoyed wearing her cadet nurse uniform, and just like the brochure stated, she "wore it proudly and wore it right." In gray and regimental red, in summer suit or winter, with snowy white blouses and shining shoes, cadet nurses made sure that hair nets were in place so hair would clear the collar. The beret insignia was pinned on the left front, and matching handbags were swung from the left shoulder. The silver Maltese cross was centered on each red epaulet for a junior cadet, and then a second cross was added to designate senior status.

On a short break while visiting Chicago, Sharon found herself in the midst of a war bond rally. She, along with other military service men and women, were called to a makeshift platform. Sharon said, "I was overwhelmed to be greeted with applause. Like the Army, the Navy, and the Marines, my cadet nurse uniform showed that I was participating in the war effort. The uniform stood for patriotism, and I was proud to show that I was serving my country."

When Sharon became a senior cadet, an opportunity arose for a field experience in a rural hospital. Sharon jumped at the chance and left for Grand Rapids, a rural town located 275 miles north of Rochester, Minnesota. In the early 1880s this area in northern Itasca County was known as the gateway to the Chippewa National Forest, the focal point in northern Minnesota for trade with the Indians. Sharon said that some took her for a French-Canadian Indian since few, if any, locals, had seen a Japanese American before. The Caucasians were mainly emigrants from southern Europe (Slavic groups), Finland, and Scandinavia. Hence the occasional "lutefisk and lefsa" were served on special days in the small 55-bed hospital. The men worked as miners in the Mesabi Iron Range, and others were loggers and farmers.

Sharon and the three Caucasian cadets were given the one available apartment in the small town. Then the nursing coordinator took her aside, explaining that the landlord of this one lone apartment did not want a "Jap" living there as his soldier son was stationed at Guadalcanal, an island in the western Pacific. Instead a deaf-mute couple opened up their home to the "Jap." Sharon said that living with the Swedish couple and their two sons gave her an insight into their handicapped condition and they enriched her life. They continue to keep in touch and are friends to this day. Sharon said, "After such a welcome it is to the credit of this town that they gave me a big send-off dinner when my experience was over."

The four senior cadets served at the Itasca County Community Hospital governed by the "Poor and Hospital Commission." The agency also ran the county home and the welfare board. Because Sharon worked this commission, a social worker drove her for health work in remote areas. Sharon loved the drives through the backwoods with her teammate, and together they checked children in one-room schoolhouses and visited invalid patients in their homes. When not on the road, Sharon assisted with home deliveries and worked on the wards of the isolated 12-bed hospital. Sharon participated in the village activities and helped decorate the small hospital at Christmas time. One of the local doctors had a party for her on her twenty-first birthday at his boathouse, and the hospital staff provided the food.

Back at St. Mary's as a senior cadet, Sharon had an opportunity to visit New York City with her friend, Ida Sakohira. The cadets stood in awe as they watched General Dwight D. Eisenhower return in triumph with a ticker-tape parade. Sharon said, "The heat of the day made no dent in our enthusiasm as we cheered and shouted. The General wore his famous happy grin, and I felt fortunate to be able to see him. It was a day I'll always remember."

After graduating from St. Mary's, Sharon returned to Seattle and began working on a nursing degree at the University of Washington. She then worked as a public health nurse and met her future husband, Ted, in church. After the arrival of three children she returned to the University of Washington for a degree in education so her hours would coincide with her school-aged boys. She was one of the first Japanese Americans to be hired by the Seattle School District and assigned to the library as a reading specialist. Once more Sharon was inspired to return to the university for a master's degree in library science. Sharon was the recipient of several awards for her work with school children.

In retrospect Sharon said that she applied the depth and breadth of two professions, that of nursing and education.

Sharon added, "The motto of St. Mary's Hospital School of Nursing was 'Enter in to learn, Go forth to serve.' Nursing with love paved my way. Those cadet nurse years were memorable."

Ida Sakohira Kawaguchi, Part 2

*What a shock when I learned that Todd [Ida's brother]
had been killed in action on the 4th of July in Italy. The
news was particularly devastating because I had not seen
Todd before his overseas assignment.*

IDA SAKOHIRA KAWAGUCHI was both sad and frightened the day she
left Gila River Relocation Camp. When it came time to load the bus,
she was in tears as she waved goodbye to her family. She was happy to
have some familiar faces on the bus to keep her company as she was
scared at being on her own and living in a distant land away from the
West Coast.

Ida arrived at St. Mary's Hospital School of Nursing in Rochester,
Minnesota, in time to start her nurse's training February 1944. Her
roommate was Sharon Tanagi Aburano (her story precedes this one).
There were seven Nisei young women in her class. Snow was a new
experience for Ida, and she had to learn how to bundle up for protection against the inclement weather. Ida lived in the nurse's dormitory in
back of the hospital, and she took the underground passageway to the
dormitory on cold, snowy days.

Three years at St. Mary's was exciting, eventful and sometimes a
traumatic time for Ida. Her first unforgettable event was the capping
ceremony, which marked the end of the probationary period and first
three months of training. She and her classmates were proud to wear
the school uniform and to participate in the beautiful candle-lighting
ceremony in which they received their caps.

Ida missed her family during holiday time and remembers a couple
who befriended the Nisei nurses. Every Christmas they invited the

Nisei cadet nurses for dinner and had a small gift for each person under the tree. Ida's most memorable vacation was traveling with Sharon Tanagi to New York City where her brother Frank had relocated and was teaching a Japanese language class. Frank showed the cadets the sights of the city.

One day Sister Antonio called Ida into her office. She inquired if there was an illness in Ida's family and explained that she had received a telegram marked with a death notice. Ida replied that she knew of no illness in her family, but had a brother who was serving with the 442 Infantry in Europe. Ida said, "What a shock when I learned that Todd had been killed in action on the 4th of July in Italy. The news was particularly devastating because I had not seen Todd before his overseas assignment."

Ida wanted to be with her family at this particular time. At first Sister Antonio said there was nothing she could do, but she later relented when Ida told her that a Memorial Service would take place at the Gila River Relocation Center. Ida's mother, Mitsuye Sakohita, received Todd's posthumous Purple Heart as so many mothers had before her. Ida's brother Harry was granted a military furlough and attended the memorial service. Mitsuye was stoic during this sad occasion, her attitude was *"shikataganai"* (it can't be helped) which gave her peace through this time of loss. Ida's mother received a letter from Dillon Meyer, Director of the WRA, which read:

> Two and a half years of war have brought heartache to many in our population. While there is little I can say today that will assuage your overwhelming grief, in the months to come you may think back upon my message with some small comfort. I am proud of your son; proud that he was an American who had the strength and courage to fight for his country in her last great crisis; proud that he was willing to give his blood as a last great measure of devotion.
>
> In a special sense, your son fought to win the war against two foes, the enemies of democracy at home who use race and ancestry to confuse and defeat the real meaning of America. It is my sorrow that he could

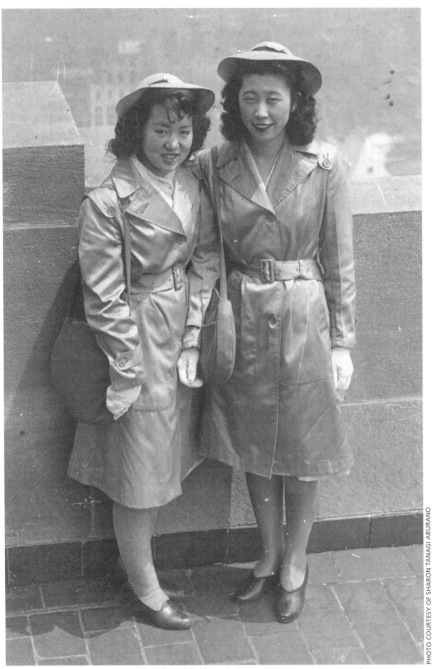

Cadet nurses Sharon Tanagi (left) and Ida Sakohira on leave in New York City.

not have lived to see his bravery, his sacrifice and his suffering bear fruit in a better world for all people.

Ida's brother Harry did not talk about his war experiences, although he received many war medals of valor. One of his battle experiences involved the rescue of the "Lost Battalion," a Texas unit who was trapped in the path of enemy lines during fierce fighting in France. There were unspeakable casualties of the 442 Infantry Unit during the rescue. When the all-Japanese American 442 Regimental Combat Team finally reached the Texas unit, they were asked, "Where are your men?" More soldiers were rescued than the remaining rescuers. The unit suffered 800 casualties to rescue 200 men. Ida's brother, Harry, was one of the few to make it out alive. Harry visited Todd's grave site in Italy before returning to the States after the war. Harry attributed his safe return from the war to a special binder with a thousand stitches that his mother had sewn for him and he wore under his clothing.

Ida wore her cadet nurse uniform when she visited the camp. The high school students were impressed and asked her to speak to the class about nursing. She gave her talk, answered questions on how to become a cadet nurse and hoped that she had steered some toward a career in nursing.

Finally Ida and her classmates had completed all of the nursing requirements in theory and practice, and graduation day arrived. The war was now over, and Ida's family had returned to their farm home in Fowler, California. Ida was excited to hear that Frank, her brother, was planning to attend her graduation ceremony. Ida said, "How proud we were when we received our diploma and school pin. Graduation from St. Mary's School of Nursing was an important day in my life."

RN

Aiko "Grace" Obata Amemiya

*We were brought closer to those who had been at war. Now
we better understood the full impact that the war had on
the men and women who served and their loved ones.*

HEARING ABOUT GOLDEN OPPORTUNITIES in America, Aiko "Grace"
Obata Amemiya's parents immigrated to the United States in the early
1900s. Her father, Tetsugoro Obata, a lawyer, and her mother, Retsu, a
home economics teacher in Japan, settled in the San Francisco Bay area.
Tetsugoro entered the insurance business and served as a correspon-
dent for a Japanese newspaper, and her mother became a homemaker.
"My parents soon learned that, like any other place, hard work was
needed in getting ahead," Grace said.

In 1930, Tetsugoro died of a heart attack, forcing the family to
adjust to a new way of life as they struggled to find prosperity. Retsu
traveled throughout ethnic communities teaching in Japanese language
schools and conducted a class after school in their home. Grace admits
that she didn't take her family's native language seriously. Grace said,
"I didn't want to spend my time after school learning how to read and
write Japanese. I was too busy playing sports." Grace excelled in softball,
tennis, track, volleyball, and basketball. Grace was valedictorian of her
high school class, and she also received the honor of outstanding girl
athlete.

Since the age of eight Grace was determined to be a nurse. She
enrolled in the University of California at Berkeley's pre-nursing
program in 1938, and she began fulfilling her dream in the fall of
1941 at the University of California School of Nursing. Pearl Harbor
abruptly changed her course. In May of 1942 Grace and her family

were interned at the Turlock Assembly Center in California and in August were moved to the Gila River Relocation Center in Arizona.

More than a year would pass before Grace could pursue her goal in life to achieve a nursing education. Throughout incarceration she served her people as a nurse aide. Grace took advantage of the training offered by Caucasian nurse supervisors, and the experience proved to be a fast way of growing up. Internment was hardest for the Issei. The mentally ill were confused, and the patients who threatened suicide had to be carefully watched. Grace said, "We saw it all—from birth to death."

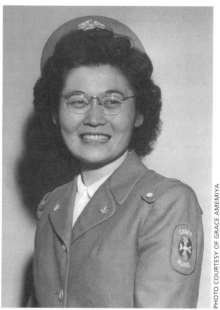

Grace Obata Amemiya, one of the first two Nisei women ever accepted for affiliation as a senior cadet in the Army Nurse Corps. (1945)

In order to leave camp, Grace had to have a job. She and a friend found work as a cook and a housekeeper for a family, and Grace began searching for a school of nursing. Many applications were sent then returned with letters stating that the quota for her "kind" had been filled. In February of 1943 Grace received the good news that St. Mary's in Rochester, Minnesota, had accepted her into the School of Nursing, making her eligible to join the U.S. Cadet Nurse Corps.

Grace elected to spend her six months at Schick General Army Hospital at Clinton, Iowa. The cadet nurses were considered officer candidates and lived in the officer quarters with strict understanding that they could not date noncommissioned soldiers. Learning to march was part of the Army protocol. Sometimes the cadet nurses' conduct necessitated a reminder that they were "in the Army" now.

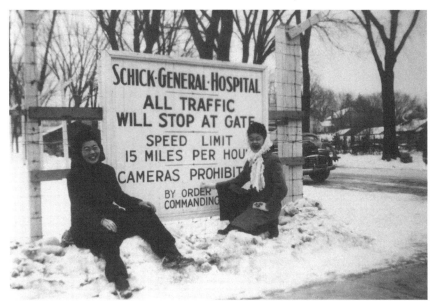

Sumi Ito, left, and Aiko "Grace" Obata, Nisei senior cadet nurses assigned to Schick General (Army) Hospital, Clinton, Iowa, 1945.

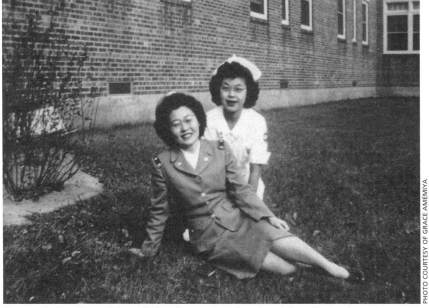

Senior Cadets Grace Obata (left in hospital uniform) and Sumiko Ito (in cadet nurse uniform) in service at Schick General (Army) Hospital, 1945.

Husband

A good friend, Minoru Amemiya, an enlisted man and sergeant in the Military Intelligence Service, planned to stop by to see Grace on his way to the Pacific war front. Grace dutifully talked to the captain in charge of the cadet nurses. Permission was granted, but Grace needed to see her soldier friend off grounds in civilian clothes. A few years later Minoru become her husband.

At Schick the cadets cared for soldiers back from the frontlines healing from war wounds and fractured bones. There were also those with broken spirits and broken minds that needed mending. Italian prisoners of war were housed at Schick and were assigned to work in the kitchen and dining halls. Grace recalls one day the Italian soldiers went on strike. Their issue? They were not served olive oil. Their verdict? The prisoners of war would receive no special privileges including their ethnic food of choice.

American servicemen who had been prisoners of war were arriving at the army hospital, and Grace served on the receiving wards. Her Army nurse captain was concerned that the G.I.'s might react to seeing an Asian face and told her to report any incident of abuse. Grace and her Nisei cadet nurse friend were required to have an escort to and from the hospital ward. Grace was moved when one of her patients offered to be her escort and security when on the hospital grounds.

One patient asked her if she was Japanese, and she replied that she was a Japanese American. Then he told her how lucky she was that she was in America, for the women in Japan were having a difficult time with the devastated war economy and all of the men gone fighting the war. The soldier told her that he had learned to eat with chopsticks when imprisoned in Japan. Grace experienced no prejudice among the returned prisoners of war. They were grateful for her nursing care and that the war was over.

The young soldiers were always playing pranks on each other. When the ambulatory patients returned from off-ground passes, often they would return to their beds to find that they had been "short-sheeted" or "water-ballooned" by fellow patients. Condoms filled with water had to be removed very carefully or the cadet nurse on duty would have to strip the wet beds and put on dry sheets.

Grace said, "We cadets who served at Schick General Army Hospital will forever be grateful for the experience of serving in a military hospital. We matured as individuals, and the experience made us a more caring and a better group of nurses. We were brought closer to those who had served in the war. Now we better understood the full impact that the war had on the men and women who had served and their loved ones. We proudly wore our uniforms, and if the war had not ended, we would have been ready to serve where needed."

(10) After the Corps

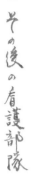

HUNDREDS OF RADIO STATIONS across America were broadcasting appeals for young women to join the U.S. Cadet Nurse Corps when suddenly, on August 14, 1945, all *end of war* broadcasts were interrupted to announce that Japan had surrendered. Recruitment for the Cadet Nurse Corps was terminated at once, but the vast nurse-training program would not close with the news of peace. Cadet nurses were supplying 80 percent of the nursing care in more than 1,000 civilian hospitals. President Harry Truman directed the Surgeon General to discontinue admission of cadet nurses to schools of nursing after October 5, 1945. Women already in the Corps would complete their training.[1]

Nisei cadet nurses heard the news of the American victory with relief and gratitude. Now their families could get back on the task of rebuilding their lives and reestablishing their homes, work, and businesses. The Japanese American cadets had shown that through perseverance they could live and succeed anywhere, now with their "lifetime education—free" (cadet nurse recruitment slogan).[2]

The U.S. government, now aware that internment had been unfair as well as unconstitutional, began taking limited steps to grant Japanese immigrants rights and privileges they had been denied before and during the war. The passage of the Walter McCarran Immigration and Nationality Act of 1952 entitled the Issei to become naturalized citizens and granted token immigration quotas to Japan and other Asian nations.[3]

In many ways, the Issei felt evacuation more severely than did their American born children, the Nisei. The older generation were in the twilight of their life careers; their average age was over 50 and such a blow as mass evacuation often brought deep-lying resentments as well as intense insecurity. A few entertained the idea of returning to Japan, and some acted upon it. But more frequently, alien parents encouraged their children to keep faith with America.[4] Nisei soldiers and nurse cadets found the Army life and the arduous cadet nurse training easier when supported by their families.

Ida Sakohira Kawaguchi said, "Some of the cadet nurses in my class accepted positions at Saint Mary's Hospital in Rochester, Minnesota, but I decided to return to our modest ranch home in Fowler, California." While many Japanese families lost their property during the internment, the Sakohira famiy was fortunate that a neighbor watched out for their land and possessions. Frank, Ida's older brother, had been hard at work remodeling. The family now had electricity, running water, an indoor bathroom, and a nice rug on the floor. Ida said, "I hardly recognized it…it was beautiful."

Ida's first employment as a registered nurse was at the Veteran's Hospital in Santa Monica, California. She was assigned to the psychiatric unit administering medications, taking part in group therapy sessions and assisting with insulin and electric shock treatments. Ida said, "It was depressing watching the war veterans with emotional problems and psychoses in the aftermath of war. We did not see many patients improve and being discharged."[5]

In the spring of 1945, Sumiko Kumabe Tanouye graduated with a bachelor's degree in nursing from the University of Colorado and the war soon ended. She sought permission to leave for her home in Hawaii and placed a request with the U.S. Army in Washington, D.C.

During the three-month waiting period she worked as a staff nurse at Colorado General Hospital in Denver.

Sumiko received classification giving her "Essential Personnel" and was granted permission to travel as a civilian on the U.S. Army troop train from Denver to San Francisco. In October 1945, she departed from the Naval Base on the converted U.S. Army troop ship, the S.S. *Monterey*, which was a former luxury liner. Other essential civilian personnel on board included nurses, laboratory technicians, teachers, and military families, all returning home after the war.

Four Caucasian recent graduate nurses, all former cadet nurses, were also aboard. The two accredited schools of nursing in Hawaii could not participate in the U.S. Cadet Nurse Corps because the territory was in the war zone. Soldiers deployed to serve with the occupation forces in Japan drilled each day on the deck. Sumiko and her cadet nurse friends enjoyed watching their maneuvers. After five days Sumiko reached her homeland of Hawaii. She took her first plane ride, an amphibian, on an inter-island flight via the Hawaiian Airlines. Sumiko said:

> The two hour plane ride to Hilo compares to 40 minutes on a commercial airliner today. But this was an improvement over the usual overnight boat ride I had experienced in the past. I was overjoyed to be with my family after being away for seven years.[6]

Yoshiko Taigawa Traynor was born in Roseville, California, in 1926 and decided on a nursing career after visiting her ailing father. After Pearl Harbor, Yoshiko and her family were interned in the Tule Lake Relocation Center in California where she graduated from high school. She was determined to find a way to get her nursing education and submitted many applications before a school of nursing would accept her.[7]

In the spring of 1944, Yoshiko entered the St. Barnabas Hospital School of Nursing in Chicago and joined the U.S. Cadet Nurse Corps. After graduation she began working in a veteran's hospital, but her ultimate goal was to join the U.S. Navy. An impossible dream? The Navy did not accept Japanese American recruits at this time. But determined

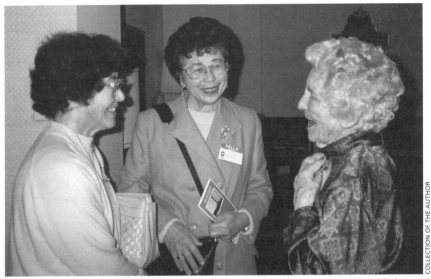

After 50 years, Stella Hoita Kato (far left) and Ida Sakohira Kawaguchi (middle) thank Lucile Petry Leone, emeritus director of the U.S. Cadet Nurse Corps, for their ticket to freedom and a lifetime education—free. San Francisco, 1994.

Yoshiko was about to make headlines in newspapers and periodicals across the country. A clipping from the national affairs section of *Time Magazine* (June 14, 1948) read as follows:

> Yoshiko Tanigawa, 22, a Nisei girl who spent 20 months at the Tule Lake detention camp during the war, was commissioned an ensign in the U.S. Navy Nurse Corps, went on duty at the Long Beach, California Naval Hospital. She is the U.S. Navy's only Japanese American officer.[8]

Yoshiko was commissioned March 3, 1948 and served as a Navy Nurse until March 9, 1950, three days after her marriage to Captain W. L. Traynor of the Marine Corps. Regulations mandated that women resign from military service after marriage. Yoshiko died March 11, 1996. She is buried in Arlington National Cemetery along with her two sons.

After the war, the changing character of the American political scene began to promote healing, renewal, and opportunities for all women, including Nisei, to expand their horizons. Suiko "Sue" Kumagai joined the Army as a diploma graduate from the Denver General Colorado Training School for Nurses in 1944. She was discharged when the war ended and remained in active reserve status. During this time she used her G.I. Bill of Rights to achieve a bachelor's degree in nursing from the University of Colorado. Sue was destined to serve as a nurse in both the country of her citizenship and the country of her ancestry.

References and Notes

[1] Federal Security Agency, *The U.S. Cadet Nurse Corps, 1943-1948*, (Public Health Service Publication No. 38, Washington, D.C.: Government Printing Office, 1950):77-78.

[2] Ibid, 30-31.

[3] Mei Nakano, *Japanese American Women: Three Generations 1890-1990*, (Berkeley, California: Mina Press Publishing, 1999):67.

[4] Robert W. O'Brien, *The College Nisei*, (Palo Alto, California: Pacific Books, 1949):44.

[5] Ida Sakohira Kawaguchi, Nisei Cadet Nurse Project, Boulder, Colorado, 19 January 1999.

[6] Sumiko Kumabe Tanouye, Nisei Cadet Nurse Project, Boulder, Colorado, 5 August 1999.

[7] Sarah Tanigawa Okado sent copies of the following newspaper articles: (1) "Japanese Girl is First of Race to Win Navy Rank," *Roseville News*, (no date); (2) "Navy Nurse Corps to Note 40th Year on May 13," *Long Beach Press-Telegram* (9 May 1949); (3) "Look Applauds...Yoshiko Tanigawa," *Look Magazine*, (no date); (4) On Worldwide News Front column, "Ensign Hosio Tanigawa," *Minneapolis Star* (31 May 1948). Nisei Cadet Nurse Project, Boulder, Colorado, 2 February 2001.

[8] "National Affairs," *Time Magazine*, 14 June 1948.

Suiko "Sue" Kumagai

I married Uncle Sam.

THE U.S. CADET NURSE CORPS...World War II...Hiroshima...
Korea...Vietnam—names we find in history books! But for Suiko "Sue"
Kumagai, they are the highlights of a nursing and military career. Sue,
a Japanese American nurse, committed her life to military nursing and
serving Uncle Sam both here and abroad, including the country of her
ancestry. Sue said she made two decisions early in life: one was that she
would not marry, and the other was to commit her career to military
nursing. She said, "I married Uncle Sam."

Sue Kumagai was born January 23, 1920 in the farming community
of McClave, Colorado. Her father came to the United States from
Japan in the early 1900s to work on the railroads. A few years later her
mother joined him. Around 70 Japanese families settled in the rich
Arkansas Valley in Colorado to engage in farm work.

Sue was the youngest of nine children. Her mother died shortly after
she was born, and her father died when she was four years old. A farm
friend who had just lost a baby raised Sue until she was four. When an
older sister, Toki, married at the age of 17, she took over the parenting
role.

In addition to going to public schools, Sue attended Japanese language school on Saturdays. When she was 19 years old, she decided to
leave the farm to join Japanese American laborers working in the citrus
groves of California. Her first job was to pack oranges and lemons, but
she didn't make much money because she was too slow. She had better
success at doing housework. Later that year she moved to Cheyenne,

Wyoming, to be near her sister and found work as a "school girl." In the 1930s intelligent, hardworking Japanese American girls and boys were in high demand by families who would give them work in exchange for a small salary, board, and room.

When Sue's employers moved to Denver, Colorado, she asked to move with them. Sue had her own basement apartment and continued her school girl work. Sue earned $8 a week and had Sundays and Thursday afternoon off. "About 20 Japanese American school girls lived in the Denver area, and we enjoyed each other's company on our day off," Sue said. "We even had our own baseball team."

One day a neighbor lady, a nurse at Denver General Hospital, asked Sue what she was going to do with her life. At that point Sue hadn't decided but knew that she needed to learn a trade so she could support herself for the rest of her life. The nurse friend suggested that Sue consider nursing, in which she could get her education by working and learning at the same time. Sue had not pondered nursing as a career. The nurse neighbor explained that the Colorado Training School based at Denver General Hospital offered a chance to learn a profession. If accepted into the program, the school would provide hospital student uniforms, room and board, and a small stipend in exchange for working on the wards while studying to be a nurse.

The nurse neighbor brought Sue an application. She found that she met all of the requirements except for chemistry. She signed up for the course through the Emily Griffith Opportunity School and went to class on her afternoon off. After completing the course, the director of nurses said, "Well, you met all of the qualifications. I guess I'll have to admit you." The director gave Sue the impression that she didn't like her.

Sue was now a full-fledged student nurse but it wouldn't be easy. This was 1941 and on December 7, the country of her ancestry bombed Pearl Harbor. Sue and three other Japanese American student nurses were called into the director's office. She told them that they could stay but they had to prove themselves. The FBI came and checked the Nisei nurse students for contraband (flashlights, cameras, and knives). Sue was determined to stay and tolerated those who called her a "Jap."

During her senior year of training, the U.S. Cadet Nurse Corps became available and Sue joined. She said that she didn't get a uniform. Only the Caucasian student nurses assigned to Fitzsimmons Army Hospital were allotted the snappy gray uniform trimmed in scarlet.

Sue visited her sister and her sister's six children who were interned at Amache, the War Relocation Center in Colorado. Sue said, "I made my sister nervous as I was defiant to the guards." Her sister asked her to include candy in the care packages which she sent on a regular basis to supplement the meager camp existence. Packages were censored before they reached the internees, and Sue's nieces and nephews never got the candy.

Sue received her diploma from the Colorado Training School in May of 1944 and took her state boards for the registered nurse license. Then she heard that graduate nurses might be drafted, so she went to the Red Cross and enlisted in the Army Nurse Corps. After completing basic training at Fort Devons, Massachusetts, Sue, a new second lieutenant was sent to Camp Edwards in Maine, which was the receiving area for war casualties. She volunteered for overseas duty, but her commanding officer wouldn't release her. Sue served 13 months, and when the war ended, the vast number of Army nurses were no longer needed. She was discharged, but remained on the active reserve status. Sue is proud of a framed letter that President Harry Truman wrote on White House stationery which reads:

> To you who answered the call of your country and served in its Armed Forces to bring about the total defeat of the enemy, I extend heartfelt thanks of a grateful nation.

Sue used her G.I. Bill of Rights to further her education in psychiatric nursing at the University of Colorado School of Nursing and received her bachelor's degree. In 1950 Sue volunteered as a civilian to serve with the Atomic Bomb Casualty Commission (ABCC). The

Field Agency was headquartered at Camp Kurihana, a former Japanese naval base near Hiroshima, Japan. The ABCC was established for the purpose of conducting long-range medical and biological research and investigating radiation effects on Hiroshima and Nagasaki survivors.

Sue witnessed the devastating effects of radiation, including babies in utero at the time of the explosion; some born with microcephaly (smaller head circumference), mental retardation, and some without skin. Studies showed that mothers with heavy irradiation had decreased male offspring. Other effects in survivors included an increase of leukemia, cataracts, epilation (loss of hair), dental problems, premature aging, and early death.

Both Sue's nursing and linguistic skills were invaluable in setting up procedures for studies by the various clinics, translating basic medical procedures into Japanese, and working with the Hiroshima Red Cross Nursing staff in the training of nurses. Sue developed rapport with the Japanese staff and conducted monthly educational meetings. Sue also taught medical surgical nursing to Japanese nurses so they could better care for the atomic war victims. The Japanese nurses were amused at Sue's dialect as her ancestors were peasant people from Northern Japan. Sue said that the speech of her people was not as refined as was the language of her students from the metropolitan areas of Japan.

In 1952 the Korean War was on, and Sue was recalled to the States for active military status. She was deployed back to Japan where she cared for American G.I.s who had been prisoners of war in Korea. She assisted in organizing the Japan Army Nurse Corps as a part of the National Police Reserve (NPR) and trained the first Japanese women to have a role in the military service. Using her bilingual and nursing skills, Sue taught 56 Japanese the six-week Japanese Army nurse basic course. She bargained with the NPR for officer's rank for the nurses. The NPR refused, and Sue said, "The best we could do for the enlisted Japanese nurses was to get them the rank of Sergeant First Class for staff nurses and for their chief nurse, the rank of Major."

After the Korean conflict, Sue, wearing boots and fatigues, served as chief nurse in the Fourth Surgical Field Hospital in Stuttgart,

Germany. But soon another war would send her back to the Pacific. During the Vietnam War she served as an assistant chief nurse in Saigon with a surgical hospital unit. In 1970 she returned to Colorado where she completed her military nurse career at Fitzsimmons Army Hospital. In 1973, Sue had achieved the rank of Colonel and retired from the Army, counting 28 years of service to Uncle Sam. She shrugs when her medals, ribbons, and citations are mentioned. She keeps them in a box and says, "Others have the same ones. You pick them up."

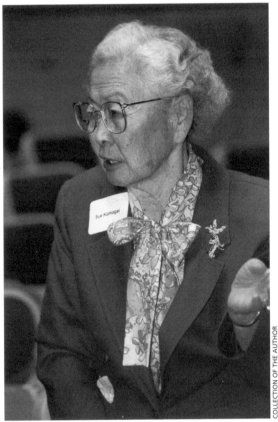

Suiko "Sue" Kumagai answers questions regarding her military career after her lecture at an International Seminar Series (2003) held by her alma mater, the University of Colorado School of Nursing.

Afterword

As the Japanese Americans began quietly slipping back into the mainstream, negative feelings in the Caucasian community gradually became more positive. The war had formally ended on September 2, 1945; Japan lay broken and defeated after the bombing of Hiroshima and Nagasaki. The Nisei men and women who had served in the war had proven their loyalty beyond question. Now the Nisei wanted to get on with their lives and to live in peace. Reflections of Nisei cadet nurses follow, beginning with Kaoru Morita Ehara:

> I have been asked by some the reason for my joining the Cadet Nurse Corps, and I have given it some serious thought. My older brother at 19 years of age had joined the 442nd Infantry and was in Italy in 1944. Why did he volunteer for the Army when his family was incarcerated? Why did I join the United States Cadet Nurse Corps? We were motivated by the deep conviction that our lives were forever American and that we could prove our loyalty by being who we were.[1]

Another Nisei nurse summarized her thoughts:

> I'm grateful to the Cadet Nurse Program, to Lucile Petry Leone for directing the program and to our government for utilizing it and for accepting me as an applicant under the circumstances. The Cadet Nurse Program was a godsend for the country and for me. I have made so many friends, and this profession has enabled me to travel to various parts of the country and to get a job anywhere I desired.[2]

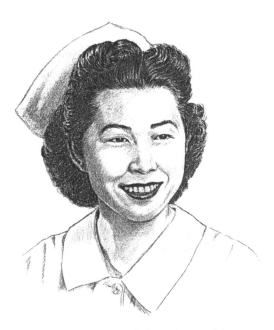

Portrait sketch of Ida Sakohira Kawaguchi, nurse
cadet in hospital uniform, 1944.

Alice Noguchi Kanagaki shared these words:

I was grateful for the education I received through this government
program that I would not have been able to afford otherwise. If we were
asked or expected to enter the armed services upon our completion, I
would have been proud to do so; after all, my three bothers were already
in the service and my joining would have been a natural progression.

Having been placed in the concentration camps was a confusing and
painful experience. Though we were never accused of any crime, I felt
guilty of being who I was, an American of Japanese descent of parents
from the country with whom we were at war. For those of us who spent
time in those concentration camps, an unexplainable feeling existed that
we shared with other Nisei. Of course this is ridiculous for having those
feelings of shame. It was difficult to talk about this time of our life for
many years.[3]

Today Aiko "Grace" Obata Amemiya is frequently asked to talk to groups of all ages regarding the incarceration of her people. Grace tells classrooms of small children about the time when she and her family had only two weeks to leave their toys, their pets, and their home. She explains to the children that they could take only two suitcases to their unknown destination. She chuckled when one small boy told her he would take his dog. Grace explained that they had to leave their pets. The little boy replied, "You could take two suitcases, couldn't you? I would put my dog in one of the suitcases and punch holes so he could breathe."

Often after her talks Grace is asked why she is not bitter. Her reply is that she would be in defeat had she let the incarceration experience take precedence in her life. Grace said, "I am not about to let something I had no control over make me bitter. You learn to do what you can do and do the best you can with whatever circumstances are thrown at you."[4]

One question has always remained for Grace: "Since they told us we were put into camp for our own protection, then why were they pointing guns in our direction?"

Another Nisei cadet nurse wrote:

In my opinion, whatever phenomenon which occurred when a large group of citizens gave up their property and were rounded-up in a detention camp would have occurred only with this generation without dire consequences. It was the time and the place. The climate was just right. The first generation of Japanese came to America seeking a better life—some were told that the streets were paved with gold. Once they realized that hard work and perseverance was the only way, they were able to start a family and build a community. At home and at school, the children were taught to be loyal to their country and to become law-abiding citizens. Another generation may not have reacted the same way; so rebellions and problems were nil, life resumed peacefully in camp—schools opened—hospitals functioned—daily life resumed.

In retrospect, does one ever ask, "Are wars, disasters, historical events planned by someone from above?" These events seem to erupt from countries the ordinary person has hardly heard of. Is the man above trying to teach us a lesson? If so, what is it? After years of combat with loss of many human lives and destruction, life goes on. Families and friends become more dear to us, even the enemies become an object of attraction and union of the young generation occurs in many instances in matrimony. Do we have to go through so much pain to achieve peace and happiness?[5]

Some women asked to participate in the Nisei Cadet Nurse Project declined, saying that they did not remember much about those times. It is understandable that for some, their memories of discrimination, evacuation, and internment are still too painful to recall. But silence does not heal. Many thanks to these Nisei women who had the courage to give us this window in time, adding to our understanding about a regrettable event in the history of our country. One of the reasons we study history is to learn from our mistakes. Forty-eight years after the mass incarceration of Japanese Americans, the Justice Department offered an apology.[6] The achievement of redress was clearly a victory for democracy.

A new national memorial—this one honors the patriotism of Japanese Americans in World War II—now occupies a tree-shaded park a few blocks from the U.S. Capitol. The National Japanese American Memorial honors the bravery of Nisei combat soldiers while recalling the shame of the U.S. internment camps that imprisoned about 110,000 people in their own country.

"Sixty years ago, we were incarcerated in these camps," said Bill Hosokawa, a longtime Denver newspaperman who is on the board of directors of the Japanese American Memorial Foundation. "We were imprisoned solely because, as they used to say, 'You picked the wrong ancestors.' Now, for the government to turn around and give us this piece of land to honor (the Japanese Americans') faith, courage, and patriotism, I think it is really tremendous. It's an overwhelming turnaround. We gave up our freedom, our homes, our friends, our businesses. This memorial is a very moving way for the government to say it's sorry."[7]

Now is the time to say *"arigato"* (thank you in Japanese) to more than 350 Nisei women who served their people in the health clinics and hospitals of the assembly and internment centers and served in the uniform of the U.S. Cadet Nurse Corps. Thanks for their service during World War II, which continued throughout their lives, and for fighting race prejudice in their quiet ways. The Japanese American women who shared their stories also taught us an important lesson in life; that of forgiveness and getting on with our lives.

Ida Sakohira Kawaguchi leaves us with this poignant message:

> It was a difficult task for me to overcome my mental block and to begin writing this paper. Once I started, the ideas, memories, and feelings flowed. My feelings of anger and despair centered around the death of my brother, Todd, who was killed in action during combat. When there were so many casualties in a unit, the unit was usually removed from the combat battle front. The 442 Infantry was not given this alternative. For this, I was bitter.
>
> As I complete this paper, I come to the realization that this life review and reminiscence involved, has helped me release the anger and negative feelings from the past. I feel that I can now work towards future goals with energy and a more positive attitude. I will be forever grateful to the U.S. Cadet Nurse Corps, which gave me the opportunity to fulfill my lifelong ambition and to contribute to the war effort.[8]

References and Notes

[1] Kaoru Morita Ehara, Nisei Cadet Nurse Project, Boulder, Colorado, 5 May 1999.

[2] Anonymous, Nisei Cadet Nurse Project, Boulder, Colorado, 6 January 2001.

[3] Alice Noguchi Kanagaki, Nisei Cadet Nurse Project, Boulder, Colorado, 16 May 2001.

[4] Jason Kristufek, "Nurse healed U.S. soldiers during W.W.II," *The Tribune*, Ames, Iowa: 29 August 2002.

[5] Anonymous, Nisei Cadet Nurse Project, Boulder, Colorado, 12 March 03.

[6] Diane Yancey, *Life in Japanese Internment Camp*, (San Diego: California: Lucent Books, 1998):95.

[7] Michael Romano, "Memorial Honors Japanese-Americans," *Rocky Mountain News*, Denver, Colorado: 22 October 1999.

[8] Ida Sakohira Kawaguchi, Nisei Cadet Nurse Project, Boulder, Colorado, 11 March 1999.

Order Form

Black Swan Mill Press
2525 Arapahoe Ave., Suite E4
PMB 534
Boulder, CO 80302 USA
thelma@cadetnurse.com

Name _____

Address _____

City _____

State _____   ZIP _____

Telephone _____

Email _____

Please send _____ copies of *Nisei Cadet Nurse of World War II: Patriotism in Spite of Prejudice*. My check is enclosed.

Pricing

    1 copy $22.50
    2-4 copies . . . . $20.25 each (10% discount)
    5-9 copies . . . . $19.00 each (15% discount)
    10 or more . . . . . . $18.00 each (20% discount)

Shipping

    For shipping within USA, please send $3.00 for the first copy and 75¢ for each additional copy. Delivery usually takes 4-7 days but can take as long as 2-3 weeks. For international shipping, please email us at thelma@cadetnurse.com

Book subtotal: $_____

Shipping: $_____

Total enclosed: $_____